STRAIGHT TALK
WITH THE
CURVY GIRLS

STRAIGHT TALK
WITH THE
CURVY GIRLS

SCOLIOSIS
Brace yourself for what you need to know

Theresa E. Mulvaney
Robin Stoltz, LCSW

Published by: Straight Talk Scoliosis, LLC
First Edition: May, 2013
Designed by Tom Emmerson, Alternative Graphic Solutions, Inc.
Cover Photo: Dana Fauth
Illustrations: Jenna Stern

ISBN: 978-0-9888231-0-5 (sc)

6070 3500
1/16

Testimonials

"Leah is an example for all of us in what it means to be courageous. Curvy Girls is a model for readers to be inspired, motivated, and empowered. Nickelodeon is proud to have been a part of bringing awareness to scoliosis. *Straight Talk* continues in the spirit of the HALO mission of helping and leading others!"

— Nick Cannon, Chairman of *TeenNick*,
Creator *TeenNick HALO Awards*,
Host of *America's Got Talent*
www.nickcannon.com

"*Straight Talk with the Curvy Girls* gives a vivid account of real life stories of young women and adolescents who have experienced the journey of living with scoliosis. Their journeys have taken them through an emotional and physical roller-coaster, depicting the mind-boggling effect of what a spine deformity can do to alter the teenage experience. Through it all, braces and surgery, these brave girls have come to embrace their curves. They dealt with it squarely, overcame it, and are now sharing their experiences to encourage girls similarly affected to be courageous and endure their treatment program. By this, they have shown that you can be bent but not broken. This is the type of support needed to foster relationships and camaraderie among girls affected with scoliosis. It is important to know that it is not the end of the world to have scoliosis. As Brooke Lyons alluded to in her books, it takes guts and courage to 'ascend the curve.'"

— Dr. Oheneba Boachie-Adjei,
Professor of Orthopaedic Surgery,
Weill Medical College of Cornell University
Attending Orthopaedic Surgeon & Chief, Scoliosis Service,
Hospital for Special Surgery
Past President, Scoliosis Research Society
Founder & President, FOCOS
www.orthofocos.org

"In *Straight Talk with the Curvy Girls*, Robin and Terry help to minimize the physical, emotional and financial burdens for scoliosis patients and families, which are often intensified by feelings of being isolated and alone. By sharing their own personal stories, young female patients and their moms give meaningful support to anyone with scoliosis and a powerful message that 'You are not alone.' In my view, this book and the Curvy Girls Support group are very valuable resources for the adolescent scoliosis community."

— Joe O'Brien, President, CEO & Patient,
National Scoliosis Foundation
www.scoliosis.org

To our daughters who brought us on this journey

For Rachel

Your dedication to bring change has inspired
this generation of kids to accept their imperfect bodies,

Proudly wear their brace outside their clothes
and speak openly about their scoliosis.

Your selflessness to help others
fueled my vision for writing this book.

Thank you for all you do to help each girl
feel less alone and more empowered.

We are all so proud of you.

To my Parents…

Who taught me the importance of family,
instilled in me that anything can be
accomplished when you put your mind to it
and who's loving spirits live within my heart

~ Theresa E. Mulvaney ~

To my children who are my purpose
My husband who is my strength
My friend whose passion drives me
To continue to make a difference.

For My Dear Leah Sara

You have always inspired me with your
fun-loving spirit and your heart, how you
see extraordinary in the ordinary, and take a
challenge and turn it into a triumph—lessons
for your life and gifts for mine.

~ Robin Stoltz ~

Never doubt that a small group of
thoughtful committed individuals can
change the world; indeed,
it's the only thing that ever has.

— Margaret Mead

Contents

Her brace
Went on
Her heart
It sank

Inside
Her
Plastic
Shell

Silently
She
Recoiled
In
Self
Despair

Her
World
Consumed
With
Worry
Overcome
With useless
Shame

A voice
Quieted
By a
Secret
Blame

A Spirit
Lost
And
Then
Reclaimed

She shouts
You will
Not
Silence
Me!

Introduction

If you have picked up this book, you must either be someone with scoliosis or you have a child with this confounding disease. You, or your child, have a spine that is growing abnormally, and you have become an unwilling participant in a race to get this core body part's growth under control ... to get it to respond to treatment, to not threaten your social or emotional lives, and to try to avoid, or at least minimize, the scope of major reconstructive spine surgery.

There are nearly seven million children, adolescents, and adults affected with idiopathic scoliosis in the United States today. Out of those seven million, children between the ages of ten and fifteen comprise the largest group affected, and the broader focus of interventions. Despite its relative commonality, there are very limited literary resources regarding this disease, and even fewer addressing the concerns that are voiced by children and parents.

Since Leah first assembled the initial group, Curvy Girls has welcomed over a hundred girls and their families who, like us, were looking everywhere for guidance and support for their child. It has been our experience that scoliosis-involved families are hungry for information. After diagnosis, they soon find themselves drowning in the hypothetical: "Why wasn't I told that?" or "If I only knew we could have done something different." In rooms separate from the Girls' meetings, parents commonly and tearfully lament over their guilt or regret for not having intervened sooner, for not pursuing the right information, or for refraining from advocating in some way on their child's behalf. These are just a few of the sentiments that are echoed over and over that became the catalyst for our writing this book.

Curvy Girls Scoliosis Support Groups was borne of thirteen-year-old Leah Stoltz's desire to connect with other girls who experienced the confusion, embarrassment, and fears that she felt while her body was growing and her spine kept curving. Leah and her group members reclaim what their deformities were threatening to take away, their sense of self-control and overall self-image. Girls, who came in thinking that they were alone in their struggle with scoliosis, connected with other girls facing similar challenges.

The monthly group discussions ranged from solving their scoliosis challenges, fashion solutions for bracing, dealing with teasing and bullying, coping with insensitive medical practitioners, and preparing for, or recovering from, spine surgery. But most importantly, Leah taught them the importance of communicating. Encouraging the girls to share their frustrations, fears, and loneliness took away the power that scoliosis had over them.

Since scoliosis is a lifelong condition, children and families need to arm themselves with knowledge and support so that they can navigate the emotional and physical challenges of this disease, as well as the health care system at large. There are many unknowns and variables that are associated with scoliosis (e.g., rate of curve progression, length and types of treatment, aggressive vs. conservative approaches) that can easily overwhelm parents and children. As consumers, we often feel dependent on health care professionals, while assuming a passive and helpless position awaiting the next appointment or exam results.

It is our aim to provide readers with encouragement and skills necessary to deal with the special challenges for scoliosis-involved families. Once empowered with information, parents' frustration and sense of powerlessness seems to dissipate. Robin's professional insight into the psychological issues of pre-adolescents and parents, together with Terry's determined call to find answers in mainstream and complementary science beyond the common "wait-and-see" approach, provide those insights and solutions.

The standard of care for scoliosis in this country—observation, bracing, or surgery—has not changed in over a hundred years. There is a gap in our health care system with regard to conservative management options. Surgical interventions have made great strides in the advancement of technique and equipment; however, there needs to be a balance. Straight Talk's goal is to fill this void so that the next generation of families affected with scoliosis will have a new, clear protocol for the standard of care. Don't we owe it to our children to pursue the safest, most effective treatment for scoliosis rather than the "wait-and-see" approach?

Prologue: Secrets

They eat away and gnaw at you. Secrets aren't healthy. Secrets develop when you think you have something to hide, something that causes you to feel embarrassment or shame. Because teens may feel embarrassed by having scoliosis or having to wear a brace, they tend to keep scoliosis and the brace a secret.

Everything begins to change during the teen years—your body, your relationships, and a sense of who you are. Cognitive capacities expand, hormones begin to affect previously rational thinking selves, and parents may no longer be experienced as a safe haven; we may have even crossed over into enemy territory. All of this is normal in the context of emerging adolescence, although it feels anything but when you are in the midst of this change.

The major developmental task of adolescence is individuation—establishing one's own identity on the road to independence—which requires teens to pull away from parents and begin to align with peers. Enter scoliosis. Bracing complicates this process, as an adolescent's sense of self can literally become distorted from wearing a brace. The brace challenges self-esteem and can leave teens in a developmental limbo, no longer fully dependent upon parents, yet in fear of rejection from peers.

Middle schoolers go to great lengths to fit in. If fitting in means denying scoliosis, then they may do just that, by refusing to talk about it or even refuse to wear the brace. Because the effects of scoliosis are not necessarily obvious to the naked eye, keeping scoliosis a secret may seem easy at first. Add a body brace into the mix, and the "secret" becomes more difficult to maintain.

"I'm ashamed of wearing a brace. I'm embarrassed to wear this clunky unattractive plastic armor around my body. If it were normal, then everyone would wear one. I'm different. I'm a freak. Better not let anyone know so they don't think I'm weird." The reality is that others will only think it's weird if you do. Seven new Curvy Girls came to a group meeting and we couldn't tell the difference between the girls wearing a brace and those that weren't. When we believe something is strange, we tend to act as if it is and our embarrassment may give away our secret. Now there are two secrets: scoliosis encased in a brace, and our shame.

Each child deals differently with the challenges of wearing a brace. We've seen a few common scenarios: some teens may refuse to wear their brace, some pretend to wear it and remove it while at school, and others dutifully wear their brace and hope no one notices. The latter is not a realistic expectation because while most braces are often well hidden under clothing, the act of lifting an arm, bending, or getting clothing caught in a chair hold the potential for exposing the "secret." The effort it takes to maintain a secret can be emotionally exhausting.

So girls, if you're embarrassed
over having to wear a brace,
you need to come up with some
good responses to, "What is that?"

One very sophisticated eleven-year-old offers this as an explanation, "I got into a sky diving accident." What does that convey? That statement says, "I am not ashamed." Because she uses humor, she demonstrates a sense of confidence. Maybe that also says not to mess with her. But this may not be your style. Just as Leah tells the Curvy Girls, you have to find your own voice. Think about what will work best for you when someone accidentally knocks into your "abs of steel."

Practice your response with a trusted friend or family member. Leah's older brother, Paul, teased her all the time about her brace. It gave her good practice! Initially, I got mad that he was making her feel badly about herself and tried to intervene. That didn't stop him. Years later, he told us that he was just trying to bring a little levity into the situation, hoping it would help her deal with kids' comments.

Deanna's bracing experience was different from most. Her friends embraced both her and her brace. She shared her secret with friends and they even named her brace. Her brace was accepted in a ceremony among her peers. Most kids are not as fortunate and may not have the support system that Deanna had with her friends. However, pretending that your brace doesn't exist wears at your self-esteem, so it's important to find a way to talk about it.

When you put so much mental energy into thinking about how to keep your brace from view or touch—no random touching, hugging, or bumping into someone in the hallway—it weighs heavy on your mind. Feeling different can be channeled into a positive direction once you speak openly about your scoliosis. Leah works on helping kids to understand that scoliosis is nothing to be ashamed of, and that if they share their "secret" they will lighten their load.

Secrets are burdensome, and shame is damaging to one's spirit.

Alyssa's dad had to drag her to her first Curvy Girls meeting. She hung her head in defeat when she walked in. No doubt she would have liked to ignore all of us. Being polite by nature and upbringing, she quietly glanced up in greeting but the sadness in her eyes broke our hearts. She didn't want to deal with her own brace, so why would she want to listen to stories about other kids' scoliosis and braces. She wanted to disown her brace, not identify with kids who wore them. At the precipice of her adolescence, she was withdrawing. Her dad made her a deal: come to a meeting this one time and she didn't have to come back. Alyssa did come back of her own volition—and she kept coming back even after she stopped wearing her brace. Alyssa comes back to share with others the lessons she learned.

The psychological impact of scoliosis and bracing on a teen is much different than on younger children. When a young child wears a brace, she may even feel proud.

One six-year-old came to her first group meeting all smiles. She couldn't wait to show us her tattooed brace. We had just finished making our introductions when she proudly pulled up her shirt to reveal multicolored butterflies adorning her Boston Brace. We oohed and aahed. She wanted to wear the brace on the outside of her shirt so everyone could see. After all, why would one want to hide those beautiful butterflies? Then there is seven-year-old Dana who joined fifteen teens and preteens for her first Curvy Girls group meeting. She listened intently to the girls as they recounted the trials and tribulations of wearing a brace, until she could take no more and announced, "I like my brace. My brace is going to help me and I want to wear it." We all need to take a lesson from the spirit of a child, yet as parents, we have all watched as our child's spirit faded into an adolescent cocoon where we are on the outside looking in. Adolescence: the time between being a dependent child and an independent adult. Here is where lessons for adulthood are learned.

More Than Their Scoliosis
More Together
Than Alone
Meet the Curvy Girls

PART I
MEMOIRS

LEAH

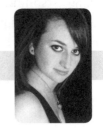

Age: 17

Braced at age 11;
Spinal fusion surgery—age 14

I started the first teen-run scoliosis support group in 2006 because I wanted to talk with other kids who were going through the same thing.

I love to dance and play golf; I enjoy reading, shopping, and traveling.

Curvy Girls has been a way for me to feel supported and give support back to others; it's never having to feel alone.

Leah's Message: Remember, it's not how big of a challenge you are given that matters, it's how you overcome it. Don't let scoliosis define or defeat you!

Coming Full Circle

Leah

Everything is spinning. Two thousand kids are shouting but I can't hear them. A tiara is placed on my head and a bouquet of red roses in my hands. "Breathe, Leah, breathe!" says Nick Cannon, the Chairman of the TeenNick Television Network, as he wraps his arm around my shoulders and puts a microphone in front of my face. I probably wouldn't believe this memory was real if there hadn't been a film crew to record every moment.

Then he announces, "I'm here to give back to someone who's been giving back her entire life." Tears start streaming down my face; I can't believe he's talking about me!

I vaguely recall being told I had scoliosis, a disease that left me with two titanium rods and 22 screws in my back. However, it was that fateful doctor's visit when I was eleven and a half years old that changed my life. I was finishing my first year of middle school when the curve in my spine began to consume my world. I wasn't happy. My body had betrayed me; I didn't feel normal. But who would be happy having to wear a back brace for twenty-two hours a day, seven days a week, for two and a half years?

MY DIAGNOSIS

I believe that I diagnosed myself. None of the school nurses or my pediatrician had noticed, but one day I was scratching around the middle of my back and something felt strange. My spine was twisted under my fingers. I asked my mom to look at it, which she did. A few days later we went for my annual check-up. During my physical exam, I showed my doctor what I had found. He said that if it was anything, it was a very minor scoliosis curve of possibly 5°. That wasn't a good enough answer for my mom. She pointed out the distinctive "S" my spinal column formed. He took out a Scoliometer and ran it down the middle of my back. Again, he said it didn't really look like much, but if we wanted, he would give us a referral to an orthopedist.

The following week when we went to see the orthopedist, Dr. Laurence Mermelstein, he said, "Definitely not 5°, probably closer to about 15°." But when I was x-rayed, the result was far from either estimate.

"This is why we take x-rays," Dr. Mermelstein explained. "Sometimes scoliosis just doesn't show."

I had two curves. My main curve in my lower back was 37° with a secondary or compensatory curve of 24° in my upper back. I was immediately thrown into a brace on June 11th, my mom's 49th birthday.

Sixth grade was probably the worst year for me. My best friend of roughly ten years dropped me cold and, at the end of that school year, I was diagnosed with scoliosis. Facing scoliosis without a best friend to talk to left me feeling extremely lonely. Then I was thrown into IT—my brace. IT was that plastic thing staring at me from my orthotist Mike Mangino's hands. How was it possible for anyone to wear IT? I felt like the world wanted to keep me down. There were two weeks left in sixth grade and I couldn't imagine how I would show up to school with IT around my body. Dr. Mike, as I liked to call him, told me that I would ease into it, so I didn't have to wear it all day until I got used to how it felt. I wore IT when I came home from school and on the weekends. Once school was over, I wore it all day to summer camp. And boy was it hot that summer! I kept it a secret. Only one other person besides my camp counselor and nurse knew about it, and that was only so she could help me take it on and off before and after swimming. I loved swimming that summer because it was my only real time out of the brace and I felt...well...normal.

The weekend after I got my brace was *the* horrid shopping trip. Trying to find clothes that would fit over the dreaded brace was an exercise in futility. I remember quite vividly being in the dressing room of Aeropostale® with my aunt, who made a special trip from Florida to take me on this shopping spree. Around me in the dressing room were clothes two sizes too big. I just could not take it any longer. I had tried on outfit after outfit and did not want to look in the mirror one more time to see how awkward I still looked.

I cried, "They don't fit. They don't look right. I can't do this! You can still see the brace. I look like a freak!" I felt completely hopeless. This was no longer my body but a body the brace formed. I continued crying as I looked at my reflection, disgusted. I soon learned that the flimsy materials that trendy clothes were made from quickly tore as a result of rubbing against the brace. Some of my new clothes were getting ruined. I needed to learn how to check the material for stiffness and thickness in order for it to endure the wear and tear of my brace.

Having to wear a plastic encasement
for hours on end, with no end in sight,
felt like the end of the world
to a twelve-year-old.

Then there was changing for gym class and fearing exposure. One of the challenges of wearing a brace to school was how I would get it off and on without anybody noticing. I could leave early from the class before, but I didn't want to call attention to myself. I ended up shamefully changing in the nurse's office supply closet or bathroom, and consequently arriving late for gym class. After gym, I did my best to change quickly back into my brace and clothes. Although the nurse never had a problem with giving me a late pass, I didn't want to call more attention to myself by walking into class late. In order to do all this, I had to get special consideration in school, which required a meeting and an IEP (individualized education plan), all of which made me feel different. I wanted to hide my brace and keep my scoliosis a secret from my secluded middle school world.

Wearing a brace changed the way I used my body. I could not bend down or move side to side. If I dropped something, I had to leave it on the floor hoping someone would pick it up for me. I was always outgoing, but out of self-consciousness I started to keep to myself.

After building up to full-time bracing, I wore my brace faithfully every day for twenty-two hours. My parents didn't even have to remind me. Two months into bracing, my parents surprised me when they said that my dad was going to take me to get a puppy. Being as responsible as I was with wearing and taking care of my brace showed them that I would be just as responsible taking care of the dog I always wanted.

SPINECOR® EXPERIENCE

A few weeks after wearing the Boston Brace, my school nurse told us she had just learned about a girl who, while braced in a soft brace called SpineCor®, had a decrease in her curve. Since a decrease in a curve when out of the brace was unheard of, my mother wanted to find out more. This was the first of numerous orthopedic consults we attended in the following years.

I was greeted with my choice of lollipops, and after looking at the x-rays we brought with us, the orthopedist told us several things. One, my curve was smaller than the 37° we were told; two, I was still not a candidate for the SpineCor® brace because it's not recommended for curves that exceed 24°; and three, there was no reason to be wearing my brace for twenty-two hours; I should only wear it for sixteen hours a day. She said that research shows that bracing at sixteen hours was just as effective as twenty-two hours. So let's see, my curve was smaller, brace time less, and I could have a lollipop of my choosing. Now this was a doctor!

Although it was not recommended, we did go for a consult with an orthotist who carried the SpineCor® brace. I took one look at all those straps and said, "No way am I wearing that!" I could never maneuver the straps in order to go to the bathroom.

We returned to Dr. Mermelstein to discuss "Lollipop Doc's" recommendations. Dr. Mermelstein stood by his original recommendation of twenty-two hours, saying that while statistics from a study showed that twenty-two hours of brace wear was no more effective than sixteen hours, this was merely an average of many brace wearers. Meaning that some kids fared better with sixteen hours and others with more, but who wanted to take the chance that I would be the one that needed the twenty-two hours. Too risky, so I continued with the twenty-two hour regime.

NEW YORK CITY

A year and a half after bracing began my primary curve had gone from 37° to 47°. Because it was a slow increase over a year's time, my orthopedist was not alarmed. If my curves remained relatively stable and my body didn't grow more, he felt satisfied that I would not need surgery. However, someone suggested to my mom that we should go to a particular orthopedist in the City for his opinion. Since this was at a renowned children's hospital, his opinion would of course be one of the best. It's a curious thing about "the best." We learned that what might be the best for one person is not necessarily what is best suited for another.

My mom and I drove into Manhattan during the holiday season when the City is quite beautiful but very cold. She promised we would go to the ballet, Swan Lake, when we were done with our appointment. My parents always did something to make a consultation special. The orthopedist at the hospital interviewed us before sending us downstairs for x-rays. We came with our own digital x-rays on a computerized disc but he said they like their own. So we waited downstairs in the bowels of the hospital for the "special" x-rays to be taken. Then we waited an hour for them to be developed before returning upstairs with them. He looked at my full-length x-rays, which were divided into three separate films and said we could consider not wearing the brace any longer. Boy, are these special x-rays! He went on to explain that research shows that bracing curves in the 40° range is less effective. Now don't get excited and throw away your braces after reading this because this too is "just a statistic." Many kids wear braces for curves that are more than 40° and can have a good result.

The next question my mom asked was that if we choose to continue with bracing, which we both agreed I should do, did he think my current brace was sufficient? He then took us across the hall and left us with the orthotist, who took one look at my brace and deemed it completely ineffective. Wearing only my underwear and a bra with a tank top they gave me, he proceeded to push and pull me into wet gauze. My mom was sitting there filling out papers and I'm standing in the middle of this very large room while a guy who I could barely understand was covering my torso in gauze to fit me for a brand new brace. To make matters worse, he was sitting in a chair with wheels and kept running over my toes. My winces were met with more pulling and pushing. Then the worst thing happened. This guy began to wrap my chest in the wet gauze. I had no idea what was going on, and neither did my mom until I tearfully called out to her. We exchanged a very confused glance. My mother insisted he stop what he was doing and bring in the doctor. We didn't even understand why they were fitting me for a new brace that was more restrictive then the first, when the doctor said I didn't even need one anymore. I refused to wear any brace that covered my chest. He reluctantly agreed to make it under my breastbone, all the while going on about how this was not the right way to do it.

From that day on, we have never gone to a doctor's appointment without asking tons of questions first. We never wanted to be in a situation that wasn't planned for. My mom and I also learned later on that the brace company was not part of the hospital but a separate company with offices closer to where I lived. So when the new brace was completed, the owner of the company brought the brace to my house.

After wearing this new brace for a couple of days, the owner met me at my follow-up visit with my own orthopedist Dr. Mermelstein who told him what needed to be adjusted. When I returned to Dr. Mermelstein with the fixed brace, he noted that it was made incorrectly; it was the exact opposite of what it should have been. This meant it was pushing where it shouldn't and not pushing where it should. Dr. Mermelstein called our original orthotist Dr. Mike, and asked that we be seen right away for a new brace fitting. Dr. Mike made up a new brace and I wore that one until I no longer wore a brace.

BREAKING THE SECRET

This secret showed no matter how hard I tried to keep it hidden. The thing about adolescent idiopathic scoliosis (AIS) is that it usually happens during middle school—a time when you worry most about fitting in. I felt embarrassed about having to wear a brace to school. Between worrying about being bumped into in the hallway, not being able to bend down, and having to change for gym class, my scoliosis was a burden. AIS is our big secret. I wanted to hide it from my world, and with the exception of my school nurse and gym teacher that was exactly what I planned to do. I told no one outside of my family until an eighth grade biology presentation.

Topics were randomly picked out of a bowl. Ms. Fitzpatrick told us there was no swapping; whatever topic we picked was ours to keep. I picked "pneumonia." I waited until the end of class and approached my teacher. I raised my shirt slightly so she could peek at my plastic torso and asked if I could report on scoliosis. Her encouragement was the turning point in my secret brace life.

On the day of the presentation, I walked into class carrying my brace in my hands and I used an overhead projector to project my x-rays on the wall in a larger-than-life image. All eyes were on me as I explained what scoliosis looked like inside and out. It wasn't until I learned how to share my "secret" that I could return to my outgoing self. Now if someone asked why I couldn't bend to pick up their pencil, I could tell them. If a kid knocked into me in the hallway, I could respond with, "Abs of steel. Feel 'em."

STARTING CURVY GIRLS

Although it is a common disorder, I found myself without anyone to whom I could relate. I was in the eighth grade when we located a support group held at a local hospital. My mother insisted it had to be for kids, but I thought otherwise. When we walked into the room filled with adults, some of whom had severe physical deformities from their scoliosis, I looked at my mother and said, "I told you so. No kids."

People shared their experiences with scoliosis that included practices no longer in effect. They spoke about medical issues that just did not pertain to me. I wished there were girls in braces to talk to so I could find out how they were dealing with this torture. I needed to find out how other girls my age talked about their scoliosis, how they wore their clothes, and how they dealt with wearing a brace in school and during the summer time. When we left the adult support group meeting, my mother admitted that I was right. I hated my brace and how it altered my life.

Why wasn't there an outlet where kids like me could express their frustration and pain?

Turning to my mom I told her, "I wish they had a group like this with kids."

My mother looked at me with wheels turning under her crazy, curly black hair. "Leah, if you want, you can make your own group." And that is exactly what I proceeded to do.

I made up flyers and brought them to my orthopedist and physical therapy offices. I wanted to create an environment for girls like me who could comfortably display their braces without being judged. I needed to give voice to those who felt as I did, alone.

On August 6th, 2006, a few weeks before my 14th birthday, the Curvy Girls Scoliosis Support Group was born. Four girls attended the first meeting. We talked about school, clothes, friends, and other problems relating to our braces. I closed the group that day with a simple yet poignant message, "We all have something to deal with that will shape who we are to become; this is ours." This is a message that I try to live by every day.

Since that first meeting, we've held monthly meetings, with typically ten to fifteen girls attending. The mission of my group is to help girls not feel the loneliness I felt and to be able to learn from each other. I want them to have access to the support that I lacked. We raise awareness in schools and in our communities, fundraise, make hospital visits, support each other through texting and phone calls, shop for brace-friendly clothing, and provide support to girls all over the world on our website. I help other girls talk about their experiences with scoliosis.

I started the group because it felt right to me. It was a simple action and I never realized how much I would be able to affect these girls. I opened my doors and my arms in order to talk to people who were going through the same situation. When strangers thank me, it's a strange feeling. It feels so surreal that I can make an impact simply by sharing my experiences. By sharing my negative experiences, I can help change theirs.

HIGH SCHOOL

I was in the ninth grade the first time I started taking my brace off during school without my parents knowing. It was such a cute outfit, and the brace really spoiled the look of it. Plus, I was in high school now! I wanted to be cool, not … lumpy. So right before first period, I went into the locker room, quickly whipped it off and stuck it in my gym locker, but this time it would wait there for six hours. I remember a feeling of paranoia that day. What if within those couple of hours, all the work I've done for the past two years got messed up? The worst was the thought that someone would discover it in the locker room and either vandalize it or give it to one of the coaches, and then my mom would find out what I had done. I also remember that no one looked at me any differently that day. Maybe I wanted a couple of people to comment on how much better I looked without the brace. When it came down to it, I guess I realized how much people really couldn't tell when I was wearing it. I only did that a couple more times because each time I had the same gnawing feeling.

SO CLOSE

We always came back to Dr. Mermelstein; we trusted him. He always explained things so that we all understood. At one of my quarterly visits, he said we could probably start talking about weaning me off of the brace in a few months. It was the best news ever! As we left the examining room, we recognized a girl we met before, Julie. She and her mom were visibly upset. They had just been told that she would have to have surgery. While her body had grown and changed, her brace remained on the floor of her closet. I asked Julie to come to our support group. As we left, my mom and I discussed how lucky I was. And then, suddenly, my "luck" changed.

Only a couple of weeks after that appointment, I noticed that the sides of my waist were no longer symmetrical. We thought it might be caused by the brace pressing in on one side more than the other. Maybe it would look different when I was out of the brace for a couple of hours. After two hours of dance class without wearing my brace, I looked in the mirror and there it was it was—my asymmetrical waist. We made another appointment with Dr. Mermelstein, and instead of weaning, this time the topic was surgery. Surgery. Yet I still had to wear my brace! I left that appointment and I was done.

When I found out that I had to have surgery after wearing the brace for two years, I just lost it. I cried a lot. It felt like I had no control over what was going on with my body anymore, and I didn't like that loss of control. My mom and I proceeded to fight about it. She wanted me to continue wearing the brace, "just in case," but I was done. That night, I hid my brace in the boiler room and went off to school for the first time in two years without it. I had struggled for long enough and I just couldn't deal with it any longer. I had to make my own decision. In fact, I made a list that day at school called, "*10 Reasons I Don't Want To Wear My Brace.*" I remember showing it to my friends and having them read it before I presented it to my mom. I—Was—Done.

⁓

But what about the group? Was I going to have to stop leading the group? I wondered how I could help them now. Wasn't the goal to avoid surgery? Had I failed? How would I be able to sit in a room of Curvy Girls, and tell them that they need to keep wearing their braces? It didn't make sense until I realized that the group was about more than just what I said to the girls; it was about being surrounded by people feeling, saying, and going through the same experiences. Even if I'm not the perfect role model for the girls, I still have things to tell them that I wish people had told me. The bottom line is that I was alone for the beginning of my bracing years, and I didn't want any other girls to have to wake up dreading getting dressed and going through school the way that I had.

No one should ever have to feel this way.

THE LAST STRAW

It was probably the first time I actually wanted to go to school. I was so done with doctor's appointments and second opinions, third opinions—and even fourth opinions—that I was literally using school as an excuse to not have to go to this "one last opinion" all the way in Brooklyn. I refused to get out of bed and into the car, so they did the only logical thing they had left to do: My gentle and generally supportive dad dragged me out of bed, hair a mess, no make-up, no glasses, and wearing raggedy pajamas. They threw me into the car, and off we went.

Before I knew it, I was sitting in the waiting room. All of these places look the same: magazines, gray walls, a couple of tattered children's books, and that toy with the different colored wires and beads. My mom was sitting next to me filling out the typical paperwork for the millionth time. It was the usual: name, d.o.b., insurance, blah, blah, blah. The silence was broken as she remarked, "It asks here, 'Have you ever been depressed?'"

I didn't even look at her when the words emerged from my mouth, "Shut up." To which she responded in that stupidly sickening and obviously fake tone, "We don't talk like that. People don't want to hear that." I was in shock. How could she really think I could care? She was fully aware that I'd rather be anywhere else than in yet another doctor's office, and I really couldn't have cared what other people might want at this point. After all, I was sitting there in my pajamas. Did I look like a person who cared? I was so tired of it all.

I had surgery June 29, 2007. As I am not one to sit still, surgery changed my lifestyle when they told me I couldn't do much physical activity for nine months to a year. Although I couldn't participate, I sat in on my dance classes and watched. It was pure torture. Instead of giving up my passions, I tried even harder. Once I was cleared to return to activities, I had to relearn how to do certain things, such as a rolling dance move or my golf swing. Not only was I weak, but my back, held together with rods and screws, was no longer familiar to me. Movement was restricted and limited. But I was determined. I took more dance classes, worked out at the gym, and did everything I could to reach my full potential. At my dance recital the following year, I performed in five challenging dance routines and was awarded Student of the Year at the dance studio I had attended since I was two and a half. My family was amazed. They remarked on how I became a better dancer now than before my surgery.

The main effect scoliosis has had on me is learning that no matter how big the setback, when I feel passionate about something and work hard enough, it can be done.

"Speech! Speech! Speech!" The 2,000-plus people in the crowd roared. I grasped the microphone in my shaking hand to make a speech I never would have imagined making. I looked over to some of the Curvy Girls who were in the audience.

"I want to thank them. They have become such a huge part of my life and I have seen so many of them grow in so many different ways. As much as they come up to me saying thank you after every meeting, what they don't understand is, how grateful I am to them."

COMING FULL CIRCLE

My scoliosis has been a journey and a struggle, with life lessons learned. The struggles could fill a novel and the tears could hydrate a desert, but the lessons learned show how there really is a light at the end of the darkest tunnel. Looking back, there's no doubt in my mind that the brace helped me become the person I am today. I have learned to embrace standing out, as I unwittingly became comfortable with my individuality. I have developed confidence to speak up, even if my ideas may not be readily accepted. My voice, once stifled by my brace, now reverberates with a message of hope and perseverance. What began as a self-help group for local teens has developed into a humanistic mission that has touched the lives of teenagers across the country, and maybe around the world.

As a result of the publicity following the 2009 TeenNick HALO— Helping and Leading Others—Awards, we opened our website www.curvygirlsscoliosis.com and Curvy Girls began to grow exponentially, both in the number of girls and families who joined our local group, as well as expanding nationally. No sooner did the show air, kids of all ages began to contact me asking how they could start a Curvy Girls group in their area. We guide them through the process. My mom doesn't want the girls to feel alone and I never want anyone to feel as I did.

After a few months, girls with scoliosis from all over the world began posting their own stories on our website. We now have thirty-six groups in twenty-eight states and four countries. But you know what amazes me the most? Every girl, no matter where they are from, says the same things, has the same worries and concerns, yet feels alone because she can't find anyone else to relate to.

Curvy Girls chapters are changing that one girl, one group, at a time.

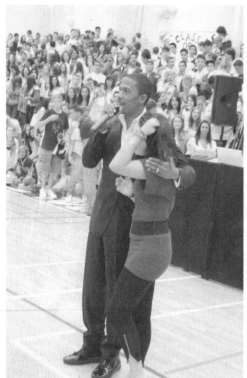

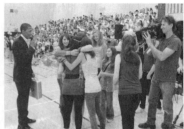

Nick Cannon surprises Leah as he brings out the Curvy Girls.

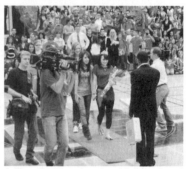

A tiara is placed on Leah's head and she is handed a bouquet of red roses before she walks the red carpet with fellow Curvy Girl Rachel Mulvaney.

Nick Cannon announces, "I'm here to give back to someone who's been giving back her entire life."

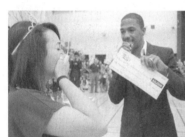

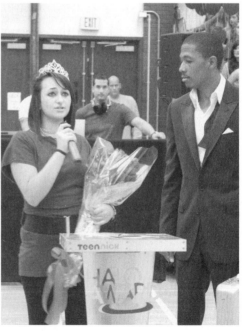

Nick Cannon hands Leah two checks—one for $10,000 for scoliosis research, and a second for $10,000 to help offset college expenses.

Leah grasped the microphone in her shaking hand to make a speech that she could never have imagined giving.

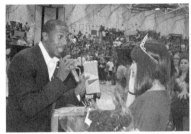

Nick Cannon surprises Leah with an all-expenses paid trip to an unknown destination to meet her secret HALO nominator.

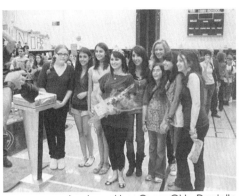

Leah and her Curvy Girls: Danielle Greenberg, Liv Mevorach, Alexis Bell, Leah Stoltz, Rachel Mulvaney, Victoria Smith, Esther Beck, Deanna Albro, and Jenna Stern.

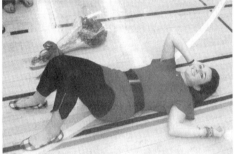

Leah is overcome with the magnitude of the event.

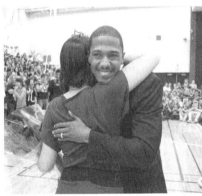

Grateful, Leah thanks Nick Cannon for everything that TeenNick has done.

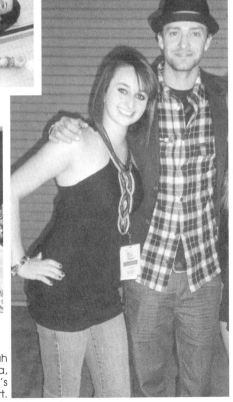

Justin Timberlake flies Leah back to Las Vegas, Nevada, for his Shriners Children's Hospital Benefit Concert.

Photo credits: Paige McCoy, Patrice Stern, Robin Stoltz

Is This Adolescence or Scoliosis?

Robin

"Start the car. When I say 'go,' you drive." Those were my husband's instructions to me for the get-away. We thought we had a solid plan. But it wasn't playing out the way we had hoped.

The commotion upstairs continued. Wild screams, "I'm not going anywhere." Leah clutched her bed sheets as her father pulled her from the bed. Leah's rescue dog, Squirt began to bark and jump in a vain effort to save his pal from her attacker. Arms flailing wildly only stayed by door jams in vain attempts to harness herself to the house. Her 200-pound once-gentle-and-kind father pries her fingers off while carrying her pajama-clad body screaming and crying down the steps and out the front door. With continued protests and a last ditch attempt to brace herself on the car door, he loads our once-sweet-and-compliant child into the back seat of the get-away car, along with the trailing bed sheets and random shoes. Who is this child? No clothing. No eye glasses. No coat. It's cold in New York in February, but we're off.

Only there's one problem. In all the confusion, her four-legged protector jumped in alongside his charge. So now, huffing and puffing, dad must remove her dog while somehow keeping our child in the car. She was either too busy kicking the back of my driver's seat to notice the opportunity for escape, or she was just too tired. Crouched down in the seat, she continued kicking and screaming well onto the Northern State Parkway and intermittently when she remembered.

What happened to our daughter? Leah doesn't leave the house without her full accoutrements of make-up and well-put-together clothes. Not unlike many adolescent girls, leaving the house entails a solid hour of closet and mirror time. We would have bet money that she would have gotten herself dressed and ready as soon as we told her we would be taking her "as is." But as any parent of a teenager can tell you, during adolescence, all bets are off! Power struggling with a teenager is a lose-lose situation. Now, add scoliosis on top and you don't know if you are coming or going. Lose-lose lose-lose.

Leah had always been a happy and cooperative child, very inquisitive and interested in going places and experiencing new things. She willingly went to all the other physician's visits, consults, and orthotists. What happened?

This is our fourth consultation and she's had enough, enough with visits to different doctors, and enough with braces. She's had it with me for making these "random" appointments, and she's had enough with feeling different. And now, she's afraid. Afraid if she has surgery, she won't be able to do what she loves most, to dance. "How long will I have to give up dance?" she asks at each consultation. This is how a young teen makes a decision about which surgeon is right for her. She cries when the doctors, nurses, and physician assistants ask her about herself, and it breaks our hearts.

Leah was diagnosed with adolescent idiopathic scoliosis toward the end of sixth grade, when she was eleven and a half years old. One evening while getting ready for bed, she came into my bedroom and said, "Feel this; my back feels weird." Leah was able to reach her arms all the way around and feel her own back. We thought she was just very flexible, but we later learned from the physical therapist that part of the problem was that she lacked stability. Was this a precursor for scoliosis? Was this the same reason her spine was too mobile? We are not aware of the definitive answer to these questions but the physical therapist believed this to be related.

Sure enough, as Leah instructed me to feel her back, I could feel a distinct curve as I ran my fingers along the upper part of her spine. Not only was I able to feel it, but now I clearly saw a curve I had never seen before. I wondered how the spine was able to bend like that; I thought the spinal column was supposed to be rigid and straight. I knew all the body's nerves ran through this area, so how was it that the spine could curve without causing a problem to the rest of the body? Maybe it was denial, the defense mechanism that runs interference for our psyche when experiencing something difficult. In my lame attempt to make sense of and normalize what I was feeling, I thought about the crown of a baby's head and how their skull bones move together as the baby grows. This must be the same type of process that happens before entering adolescence. I figured that as soon as the body caught up to the spine, the spinal column would surely straighten.

At her annual check-up that weekend, we pointed out our concerns about Leah's spine. The pediatrician said that while it wasn't significant, we could see an orthopedist if I was concerned. I made an appointment for the next day.

Upon examining Leah, the orthopedist also initially thought the curve was minor (approximately 15°), but the x-rays showed otherwise. Leah hid her curve "nicely." Not only wasn't it obvious to the untrained eye, it apparently wasn't visible to the trained eye. Leah's scoliosis was completely missed during the school scoliosis screening only five months prior. X-rays revealed that her primary curve was 37°, with a secondary compensatory curve of 26°. She gave the appearance of being balanced because her top and bottom were twisted in opposing directions.

At the time of Leah's diagnosis and bracing, my husband, Mike, was in the hospital under quarantine for radioactive treatment of thyroid cancer. He didn't even know Leah had been diagnosed with scoliosis because there was no way to reach him. I remember Dr. Mermelstein's calm and kindness; just like Leah's dad who never panicked. He was reassuring and direct while he explained the course of treatment for a 37° curve.

Later that same day, Leah was fitted for a back brace that she would work up to wearing twenty-two hours a day, seven days a week for a yet to-be-determined period of time. Her Risser measured zero at bracing, which meant that her growth plates were fully open. The trick now was to keep her spine from further curving while her growth continued. This posed an ironic twist for a mother: wanting your child to grow quickly, at a time when what I also wanted was to hold onto the innocence of her childhood. I felt as if I was being cheated.

Leah appeared to take this new information in stride. When we picked up her new brace the following week, I watched for her expression. She didn't seem upset so I kept my demeanor calm. I didn't want to alarm her to the strangeness of what I was seeing: a large plastic contraption that she would have to put around her developing body for two years! I couldn't fathom how she would be able to do this. The whole concept seemed archaic to me. Thoughts ran through my mind, "How would she ever wear something so large? Was she really going to agree to wear it? Maybe she should just skip to the surgery since that is where this may end up anyway." It seemed insurmountable, but since kids tend to follow their parents' lead, I thought it best to keep my own feelings in check and watch for her reaction. She would have enough of her own feelings to deal with; she shouldn't have to take on mine.

It wasn't until two days after we picked up the brace that I heard crying in her room. She couldn't find anything to wear that fit over her brace. We would have to go shopping. When she couldn't even find something to wear to go shopping, her crying and sense of despair grew. She cried that she just wanted to have the surgery. I couldn't imagine how we were going to find stylish clothes to go over this contraption. My heart sunk inside for her. Because kids at her age are influenced by what their peers think, my biggest worry was that someone would say something to embarrass her and she wouldn't know how to respond.

> I prayed she had the strength to know
> that the brace did not define her.

We made up scenarios about what she could say if someone asked about her brace. She only had one week of school remaining before summer vacation. She'd have the whole summer to get used to it. I wanted her to feel stronger about herself before she had to face her peers. Initially, Leah tried her best to disguise her brace but would eventually find that the best way to deal with it was to come right out and talk about it. This way, there is no secret worry about being caught off guard.

I have a coping strategy that helps me keep perspective when I feel overwhelmed. I tell myself, "Short of life-threatening, I can deal with anything." I couldn't fix what was happening to Leah. I couldn't stop it or protect her from the reality of it, but what I could do was support her and help her to develop strength; strength that could serve her through life's many challenges. I learned from my own childhood challenges and in my profession from my clients, that it is the resilience of a person that counts the most in the face of adversity. We are always faced with challenges, but if we teach our children that they can bounce back, we give them a sense of confidence and self-reliance. Leah says it best when she tells Curvy Girls, "Everyone has something they have to deal with, and this is ours."

When Mike and I saw how diligent Leah was with wearing and taking care of her brace, we rewarded her with a long awaited dog. Well, he wasn't exactly the puppy that Leah had in mind when they ventured off on their search, but Mike knew that this nervous, depressed dog needed a home. Squirt attached himself to Leah and only Leah. He would wait by her bedroom door all day for her to return home from school. He even has a crooked tail, just like her back.

Leah wore her brace faithfully for the first year, yet her main curve increased by ten degrees, measuring at 47°. Because the change was gradual, taking place over a year's time, our orthopedist was not concerned. We would wait and see if it stabilized. Over the following year, it did indeed stabilize at around the 50° point, and cosmetically she still did not look compromised. Leah didn't have the typical shoulder protrusion, which was the telltale sign of scoliosis. She looked balanced, and her body hid her curve.

As time progressed, so did adolescence. While we were in the thick of things, it was difficult to distinguish between adolescent defiance and frustration with having to wear a body brace. The ramifications of scoliosis seemed to propel her full force into adolescent angst.

She stopped hugging me. Leah seemed angry with me all the time. That is, until Sunday when it was time for our support group and her whole demeanor towards me would change. During a joint parent-teen Curvy Girls group session, she sat herself on my lap and related to me as if she did this all the time. Somehow it was safe. She was in control of her life on those Sundays, and not the victim to her scoliosis. When the meeting ended, she'd return to her pattern of feigned indifference until the following month.

Quietly, she tortured herself, hiding her thoughts and feelings behind a facade of indifference. One day after a night of nasty fighting,

I picked Leah up from school and asked her how she felt about the night before. Her response was, in no uncertain terms, "I don't do feelings." Ah, yes, why would she "do feelings" when both her dad and I are social workers. That is what we "do" for a living—feelings. What better way to separate and establish her own identity but to not "do" what we "do." And so her conundrum: Share my feelings with my parents or stuff my feelings and pretend that I don't care.

At our two-year check-up, the orthopedist said we could anticipate a plan for brace weaning at the next visit. With relief and celebration, we readied to leave the office, when we spotted another fourteen-year-old girl and her mother. Their expressions were not the same as ours. The girl's eyes were red from crying and the mother looked stunned. Their news was quite different. Leah and I stayed to talk with them. We offered comfort, and exchanged phone numbers and email addresses. Her surgery was scheduled to be in three months. Leah invited her to the support group, and Julie came with her mother. When we left the office, I told Leah, "There by the grace of God, go us." You just never know. But Leah reminded me, "She didn't wear her brace." She hated it and refused to wear it. It sat on the floor of her closet.

Well, that made sense. The formula was simple:

Wear your brace = no surgery. Don't wear it = surgery.

Or so we thought, until two weeks later.

"My waist is not even," Leah exclaimed.

(Again, denial.) "Maybe, it's from the brace," I responded.

Two days later, after being out of her brace for two hours while in dance, Leah again pointed out, "Look at it now." There it was, plain to see. One side of her waist was almost perfectly straight, while the other showed what I thought must be her newly developing waistline.

Within a few days time, back to the orthopedist we went. This time we were not as lucky. As he studied her waist, we realized it was the defining moment. Because her curve was in the lumbar region of her body, when her body developed and her waist slimmed, the scoliosis showed itself.

After two-plus years of wearing her brace, Leah was told she needed surgery. Listening to your child sob "Why me?" alone in her bedroom was heart-wrenching. Leah would have her brace/scoliosis meltdowns periodically, usually in the shower. Ultimately, she would emerge relieved. This time I could hear her dog, Squirt, whimpering outside the bathroom door. When I got closer, I could hear her angry sobs, "I wore my brace for nothing."

Leah's acting out became almost unbearable once she knew that she needed surgery. She was angry and felt as if the years spent in a brace were for naught, even though wearing the brace for those two critical years ultimately enabled her to have a better surgical outcome.

Leah saw surgery as a personal failure. She wondered how she could lead the group when she had "failed." In her mind, at least, her body had failed her and she would now fail the group of girls she wanted to support. She was surprised when I reminded her that the support group she began was not just about her giving to others. Other people needed to be able to give to her as well, to be able to offer her what she had given them. She didn't have to be the strong one or have all the answers all the time; she too could cry and feel scared. She seemed satisfied and continued with the group.

The last Curvy Girls group meeting before Leah's surgery was not held at our house, as it usually was. Instead, Curvy Girl Rachel Mulvaney with her mom, Terry, wanted us to be guests at their home. They wanted to thank Leah for all that she had done. They celebrated Leah that day. The girls bought Leah gifts useful for her hospital stay. There were fun, colored leg rolls and soft coughing pillows for after surgery, a journal to keep track of the "f" word (feelings). When I left that day, I too had learned the true meaning of support.

From the very onset, we felt confident with our orthopedist. But when it came time for surgery, we worried about where we should have it done. We were too close to Manhattan not to consider the options there. Mike and I kept saying, "You don't know what you don't know." We had to go and find out everything we didn't know, so we could feel like we knew even less. Our search into The City began. At our first encounter with "The Office with the Attitude," we were told surgery is done at 40° and the oh-so-sensitive physician assistant proceeded to tell Leah that the brace she wore for two years was "useless" compared to the one that they make. Great message!

Then we had another consult with a surgeon who authored one of the few books written on scoliosis. What was most baffling was the difference in the "expert" opinions. Each one had something different to say, which accounted for the final crazy-parent-drags-pajama-clad-child-to-Brooklyn visit. Our final and last consult was more consistent with what we heard from our own orthopedist. How were we to make sense of all the information? Should we have surgery? If so, when and with whom?

In the end, it was our own orthopedist who helped us sort through all the information we gathered and make sense of the differing opinions. He spent a couple of hours with us after the office closed, sitting at the computer, showing x-rays of varying surgical procedures, teaching, and answering every last one of our questions. He taught us that sometimes medicine is more of an art than a science. When we left, we knew he was to be our artist. He is brilliant, talented, and kind, and he leaves his ego at the door. Ultimately, the time Leah spent with Dr. Mermelstein helped her come to terms with having surgery sooner rather than later.

The local Long Island hospital where Leah had surgery, Good Samaritan Hospital, was a superior experience, a gem in our own backyard. When all was said and done, Leah was happy with the outcome of her surgery. She is pleased with how her body looks and proud of the scar that runs almost the full length of her back. The first day back to school after surgery, she wore a halter-top that her dad thought too revealing. But we decided that if she was willing to "expose" her scar, she could wear that shirt. She returned to dance much sooner than she thought and now her behavior is relatively normal. That is to say, if you consider adolescence a time of normalcy!

⌒

Leah has since finished her bracing, and surgery is literally "behind" her. Today, as a young adult, she has taken to working through issues related to how wearing a back brace and having major spine surgery made her feel about her body. Along the way, Leah learned that she wasn't alone, that she could positively impact her own life circumstances, could speak up for herself—and teach others to do the same. Perhaps more importantly, she learned that she could take control over her own body and assert herself even in uncomfortable situations. Scoliosis presented her with challenges but afforded her these many gifts.

Our relationship has been a dance of sorts, around her scoliosis and through her adolescence. We haven't yet emerged, but I believe we are getting closer. From Leah's perspective, scoliosis destroyed our relationship; from mine, the support group helped bring us back together.

RACHEL

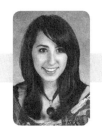

Age: 14

Braced at age 11

I enjoy watching old Hollywood films and learning about American History. I love the Beatles' music. I also love studying the histories behind fashion icons like Coco Chanel, Bobby Valentino, and Christian Dior.

Curvy Girls means unconditional support. Whether it was how we felt or what we said, we were never judged; we have total acceptance among one another. My goal today is to give back what I was given, and have the ability to listen and help others with the challenges they might face with scoliosis.

Rachel's Message: It's never too late to take back control over your body.

I Wouldn't Change a Thing

Rachel and Terry

SCHOOL SCREENING

Rachel: I was nine years old, and in the third grade, when my class was called down to the nurse's office for a scoliosis test. I watched as five or six kids ahead of me got tested. The only thing they had to do was lift up their shirt, bend forward, and leave with a lollipop, which put a smile on everyone's face. Unlike them, I left with a puzzled face because my exam was strangely different. Once my shirt was lifted and I bent forward, the nurse gasped. I had no idea what was going on. The doctor asked me to stand up straight, bend forward again, rotate to the left, and then to the right. He examined my back by feeling the direction of my spinal column. I was then asked to sit back down and let the rest of the class finish their scoliosis test. After my second examination, the nurse handed me a note to give to my mom. I didn't have the slightest clue at that time as to the challenges I would soon face. When I got home that day, I gave my mom the note and she too lifted up my shirt. It was a relief to not hear a gasp come from her.

Mom: Rachel is my fourth and last child, and this was the first time scoliosis was introduced to my family as a possible threat. I had little understanding of this disease, which is why I felt uncomfortable when I received a call from the school nurse that day. She was informing me that Rachel would be coming home with a notice stating that she failed her scoliosis screening. With a touch of sensitive concern in her voice, she advised me to make an appointment with the pediatrician as soon as possible, in order to either confirm or deny the school's findings.

I immediately called my pediatrician's office, and in the middle of my unusually long explanation as to why I needed an appointment as soon as possible, the office assistant interjected, "The school nurses are never right. We get kids all the time who fail the school scoliosis screening and pass our evaluation. There's absolutely no need to worry." I was comforted by her words, so we set an appointment for the following week.

When Rachel came home she presented me with the nurse's notice; I immediately felt a twinge of anxiety. "Rachel, can I see your back?" I asked her. Without hesitation, she lifted the back of her shirt and bent over. I stared at her back and ran my fingers up and down her spine for some time, trying to see or feel a curve, but her back seemed straight to me. My own observations, plus the comment from the assistant in the pediatrician's office, prompted me to think that this was just some miscalculation that would be corrected in a week.

On the day of the appointment, I was calm and confident. This was just a formality that would be over in a few minutes, and then we would go on as if nothing happened. My state of mind quickly changed after the pediatrician confirmed the school's findings. "Rachel has a curve of about 15°." He wanted Rachel to immediately see a pediatric orthopedic physician specializing in scoliosis. I went from blissful ignorance to panic.

I repeated silently to myself, "What did that mean?" As I stumbled with my thoughts, I knew I needed to pull myself together and start asking questions.

"What does it mean that her curve is 15°? Is that serious? What is a normal curve?"

The physician responded, "A curve that is 0° to 10° is considered to be within the normal range."

"Ok, that's not too bad; she's only off by 5°," I thought.

The doctor then asked, "Has Rachel begun to menstruate?"

I was taken aback. I could not understand why Rachel's menstruation was a matter for questioning at that moment. It was as though the doctor read my mind and immediately continued, "Girls will continue to grow for twelve- to eighteen-months after they begin to menstruate. A close monitoring will be necessary since Rachel has years left of growth."

By the end of our visit, we scheduled a consultation with an orthopedic specialist. Determined to be better prepared for the next appointment, I decided to give myself a quick education about this disease by way of my favorite Internet search engine—Google. My computer screen was instantly flooded with all kinds of information. But I was not at all ready when early in my search I was viewing images of the most severe scoliosis cases—zigzagged backs that took on the shape of the letter "S" and others which curved to either the extreme left or right side. Emotionally drained, I closed the web page and decided to get educated by the professionals, and not the Internet.

MEETING THE LOLLIPOP DOCTOR

Rachel: The first time I met my orthopedic doctor I liked her. She made a great first impression, as she greeted me with a handful of colorful lollipops for me to choose from. She made talking to her very easy. She asked me a series of questions such as, "How do you like school?" and "What kinds of activities do you like to do?" I told her all about my teachers and how much I loved to dance. She also lifted up my shirt and kept admiring how flexible I was. We were told to come back in six months for new x-rays.

Mom: Rachel's orthopedic physician was younger than we expected, warm, and very friendly. More importantly, I could tell that Rachel was comfortable because she was quickly engaged in conversation with her. Impressed with Rachel's flexibility, she encouraged her to continue to be physically active, as this would help with her condition. She confirmed that Rachel had idiopathic scoliosis with a curve of 16°; however, we were relieved to learn that no treatment was required unless her curve approached the 25° mark. In order to monitor the progression of the curve, Rachel needed to come back in six months for a follow-up visit and a new set of x-rays. Unfortunately, when we returned for this appointment, we learned that the doctor's office no longer accepted our medical insurance. We did our best to challenge their information, but were unsuccessful. The receptionist apologized for the miscommunication; they were under the impression that we had been contacted. So began my search for a new orthopedic specialist.

Several weeks later, I found a new doctor in our health plan; however, his first appointment wasn't for six months, which would have made Rachel's follow-up a full year later. Determined to get an earlier appointment with another specialist, I declined. This turned out to be a decision I would later regret. Unconsciously, I was allowing Rachel's scoliosis to take the back burner while I let other seemingly more serious problems take priority in our lives.

Rachel: During this time there was a lot going on with my family. We moved into a new house, I went to a new school, and my grandfather became very sick. Within six months of moving, my grandfather, who I was very close to, passed away on my sister's birthday. It was the saddest day of my life and it seemed to only get worse. Six weeks later, my mother, sister, and I witnessed our beloved dog, Honey, get hit by a car and die. Nothing seemed to go right. I tried to tell my mom I had back pain, but I could tell she wasn't taking what I said seriously. It was as if there was a black cloud over our family. My grandmother was depressed from losing her husband, and my sister was out of school for nearly three months with a severe case of mononucleosis. My back pain persisted, but I kept it to myself. I didn't want to add more stress onto my mom.

One evening, my pain became too obvious to hide. I couldn't walk without discomfort and I finally asked my mom to rub my back. It was then she realized that the pain I had complained about was real.

Mom: It felt as if a thousand things were happening at once. Up until Rachel's diagnosis, life might have been crazy, but somehow I was able to balance it all. Then, in an instant, everything changed. The six months following the death of my father was an emphatic testament of the old saying, "When it rains, it pours." It was during this period when Rachel began to complain of back pain. As horrible as it sounds, I couldn't deal with it, not after losing my dad, and having to face a long list of adversities that seemed to pile up aggressively against my family. I am embarrassed to admit that I ignored my daughter's complaints, convincing myself that her back pain was no big deal, and that she just wanted attention.

It wasn't until weeks later that I noticed she was bent forward holding her left hand on her lower back. She looked up at me and said that her back was killing her, could I please rub it. I motioned her to come over to me and she lay forward on my lap. I was dumbfounded as I pulled her top up, and frightened at what I saw.

The lower left side protruded like a small hump, while the right side of her back appeared normal. While I continued to rub her back, I couldn't help but notice an unmistakable bend in her spinal column that pulled to her right. The entire right side of her back seemed to bulge out. Her right rib cage protruded and appeared disproportionate to the other side. The center and left side appeared to be sunken in comparison to the protruding side.

I felt physically sick as I realized that this child was not seeking attention; she was in pain. I felt like the world's worst mother!

THE TURTLE SHELL

Rachel: The next thing I knew, I was back to see the "Lollipop Doctor." It was at this office visit that we learned my curve had gone from 16° to 35°. I heard the doctor tell my mom that I needed to be braced immediately. She further explained that I had to wear this back brace for sixteen hours a day for the next two- to three-years. I thought she was crazy, especially when she started to describe what the brace looked like, and how it would fit my body.

The doctor said, "It's like being in a very tight turtle shell."

I couldn't help but cry. I remember my mother just holding me and saying, "Rachel you can do this. Don't cry. Everything will be okay."

Mom: My eyes swelled with tears and my lips began to quiver, as I silently began to blame myself for this entire mess I put my daughter in. I tried to speak without breaking down, as I watched Rachel try to process what all this meant. In a very shaky voice, I managed to ask, "How can your estimation be either two or three years?"

"Well, I don't know for sure, it depends on how much growing she has left to do. She hasn't begun to menstruate, and the growth plate in her pelvis is at a zero," she explained.

"Okay, well what number will tell you that she's done growing?"

"When she reaches a Risser 5, her growing is complete. This concerns me because we usually discuss corrective surgery when her curve hits the 40° mark," she concluded.

A million things were rushing through my mind, but the most important was figuring out a way to help Rachel get through whatever might lie ahead. Before we left, we were given a list of prosthetic offices that made the Boston Brace. On the way home, Rachel began to cry uncontrollably and I tried to hide the tears rolling down my face.

LET'S STRAP THEM IN

Rachel: Within forty-eight hours, I was being fitted for my first brace, the worst experience of my life. I never knew a medical professional could be so rude and inconsiderate of a child's pain. I was hysterical crying and he never once asked, "What's the matter?" It was my mother who asked, "Why is she crying like this?"

His answer was, "She's not used to wearing a brace yet."

I gave him a dirty look and said, "No, I feel like I can't breathe. Please take it off!" More tears came down my cheeks and I said again, "Take it off!"

And all he said to me was, "Suck in your stomach and hold your breath," as he yanked each strap as tight as possible.

Mom: Having my child fitted for a back brace for the first time by a local orthotist was extremely foreign to me. I knew nothing about this process. The orthotist warned me how much my child would cry and complain regarding the discomfort of the brace. This translated to mean that I needed to be especially strong. I reminded myself that if Rachel was sick and had to take a horrible tasting medication in order to get well, even if she cried, I would make sure she would swallow it. I watched as they roughly maneuvered her, measured, and prodded her with their instruments. No matter how strong I told myself I had to be, my heart was breaking watching Rachel's eyes well up with tears. It was the worst feeling in the world because I felt like I wasn't allowed to say anything. They put the brace on so tight that Rachel immediately began to cry.

To be honest, I was scared and intimidated to speak up.

Rachel: I couldn't wait to get out of that office, and when we left, I ripped the straps right off. Finally, I could breathe. I thought these people were out of their minds to think I'm going to wear this contraption for sixteen hours a day. For me personally, I think every doctor in the field of scoliosis should be fitted for a back brace and wear it for one week, sixteen to twenty-three hours a day. What better way to understand what it feels like to be strapped and pulled so tight; like a boa constrictor holding its prey.

My parents kept saying that everything would be okay, but the only thought I had was "easier said than done."

> No one knew the emotional
> and physical pain I was
> going through, let alone how scared
> and alone I truly felt.

All I kept doing was going over everything in my head. My mind was filled with anger, fear, and frustration. I was angry that I had to wear this horrible brace, scared that I might not be able to find clothes to hide this brace from the world, and frustrated because there were no guarantees. You see, I could do everything they told me, and still have to face surgery one day. They just didn't get it.

Mom: The next day we met back at the doctor's office for another set of x-rays, but this time she was to be x-rayed wearing the brace in order to see how well the brace was correcting her curve. She measured 35° without a brace, and 25° with the brace on. Again, not ever thinking an expert would not know what they're doing, I believed this was good; the brace was doing its job no matter what discomfort Rachel was experiencing. Wrong. I would later learn that bracing shouldn't cause that much pain.

As the weeks progressed, so did Rachel's pain. I continued to bring her back to the doctor, and though they never called her a liar, they reminded me that scoliosis is a disease that is not associated with pain. I knew my daughter wasn't lying. If she said she was in pain, then she was in pain. They gave her anti-inflammatory medications, but that didn't work. They ordered an MRI but that could not be completed, because no one realized that Rachel's orthodontic braces created a terrible pulling sensation as the magnets in the machine traveled further towards her upper body. My frustrations only escalated. I wasn't sure whom to be angrier with, her doctor who ordered the test, or the technician who clearly did not read that there was metal in her mouth.

BEING POWERLESS

Rachel: To be honest, I think the hardest part of the entire journey was just feeling angry all the time. I hated how this feeling took control of me. Whenever my mom tried to say something supportive, I didn't want to hear it; I didn't care. She didn't get it, no one did. Everything was changing so quickly in my life and I felt like I had no control. I was totally powerless.

To make matters worse, I learned that my father allowed my teacher to tell my entire class that I had scoliosis and that I would have to wear a back brace to school every day. What was my dad thinking, or my teacher? Why would they believe that kids in the fifth grade would be mature enough to handle my diagnosis of scoliosis? I guess now I realize they were trying to help, but I wish someone back then had asked me my opinion.

Every day, wearing this brace to school became harder because everyone knew. Everyone wanted to see it, touch it, and yes, some of the girls wanted to try it on. I was so angry at my mom for making me wear this stupid brace to school. She would say she understood, but she didn't. She wasn't living, breathing, eating, or sleeping in this thing; I was.

Mom: When no answers were found, I observed my once active outgoing daughter become very withdrawn, no longer going out or interacting with her friends. Since we were just bracing after school in the beginning, she would literally come home, do her homework, and then go to sleep on either the couch or her bed for hours. When this routine of hers continued for weeks, I called my pediatrician's office for an exam. I truly began to fear that Rachel had a serious medical condition since she was so lethargic. The pediatrician listened to the symptoms and then asked Rachel if there been any recent changes in her life. She mentioned that her grandfather died, we had lost our family dog, and that she just found out she has to wear this brace for sixteen hours a day (which she demonstrated by knocking on her stomach) because of her scoliosis.

The doctor then asked Rachel, "How's the bracing going?"

Rachel responded in a low fragile voice, "Okay, I guess."

He began to ask more questions and we soon learned that years ago his daughter was also diagnosed with scoliosis. This seemed to help Rachel open up, and I began to hear all the emotional and physical pain she had been holding in. The pediatrician listened.

He looked at me and said, "I could order every test but I truly believe Rachel is suffering from depression."

As soon as he said those words, I looked over at Rachel to see her head nodding up and down as tears were silently running down her face. It was at that moment that I realized the impact the brace was having on her life.

Rachel: It's hard to explain how everything I was feeling was not me. The girl who was once so outgoing and happy was quickly disappearing. The colors began to fade away as I felt myself falling into this dark hole. Sleep became my great escape. I felt that if I were sleeping, it would be fewer hours awake in the brace.

Mom: I brought Rachel back to our orthopedist to share my concerns and asked her to look at the brace. After she examined the brace, she could see the areas that were causing Rachel's pain and bruises. She suggested bringing the brace back to the orthotist for adjustments. We went back to this orthotist three more times and, unfortunately, the only thing that seemed to change was that the owner of the company became involved. I'm not sure why, but I actually believed that they thought we would be impressed by the owner offering his expertise. But we were not.

Rachel: With each visit back to the orthotist, nothing ever changed. The orthotist was always cold and insensitive and I hated his condescending tone when he spoke to me; he only made me cry more.

Mom: "This cannot be a normal reaction to being fitted for a brace," I said to the orthotist.

He didn't respond. Was he ignoring me? Rachel continued to cry and I lost it. I ordered him to just take the brace off of her, and I insisted that something was wrong.

The last comment he made was, "She'll be fine. This is still an adjustment period she is going through."

By now Rachel was hysterical, and we left.

Rachel: I had no choice but to continue to wear my suit of armor under my clothes. School was almost over and I was excited that I didn't have to deal with the dressing issue much longer. The only other activities that made me somewhat happy were my dance classes; there I was able to be brace-free for the hour. Unfortunately, as my back pain increased, dancing was becoming less enjoyable. After nine years of dance, I finally just gave it up.

I think one of the worst experiences I had with my back brace was a trip to the emergency room. Sharp pains shooting down my right leg and abdomen were so intense I wasn't even able to walk up stairs.

Mom: On the initial emergency room exams, Rachel was symptomatic for an inflamed appendix. As each emergency doctor gently pressed down on the lower right side of her abdomen, she jumped with pain. One of the attending physicians noticed Rachel's deep red marks toward the lower right side of her abdomen where her pain was located. He asked Rachel to show him how she wears the brace.

Rachel: Initially, I had no idea why the emergency room doctors were asking to see my back brace or have me put it on for them. Once on, I immediately flinched with pain as the bottom of the brace dug into my right lower abdomen. They observed the bruises and how it lined up right next to where my brace was digging into me and causing pain. A light bulb went on for one specific doctor when he realized my appendix was literally bruised by my back brace.

Mom: Having the emergency room doctor conclude that her brace was bruising her appendix made me crazy. Rachel was instructed to stop wearing the brace until changes were made to the brace and the inflammation subsided. As Rachel proceeded to get changed, I couldn't help but become furious. We trusted the "experts" to help our daughter, but it was apparent now that they didn't know what they were doing. The next day my husband returned their useless piece of plastic.

Rachel: I was out of the brace for several weeks until my abdomen healed. When I finally resumed bracing, my parents found a much more professional office to work with. My new orthotist, Steve Mullins, explained that bracing is never comfortable, but what he promised to do was make it as tolerable as possible. This experience was nothing like what I went through four months earlier. It was like we were working together. I told him where it hurt, and wherever he could, he made adjustments. I left there much happier than I ever expected. I was wearing the brace and not crying. I actually felt confident for the first time that I might be able to do this.

Mom: Watching Rachel being refitted for a new brace with no tears was amazing. The difference in her care was like night and day. When the new brace was completed she said it was tight, but she could still breathe. Within a few days, Rachel was able to meet her required sixteen hours of bracing a day. As an extra bonus, when she was re-x-rayed in her new brace, her curve decreased to 18°! This was a remarkable improvement from the previous brace, where the orthotist was only able to decrease her curve to 25°.

THEY DON'T UNDERSTAND

Rachel: My bracing problems disappeared, however my back pain never went away. My follow-up appointments were supposed to be every six months, but since I was still in so much back pain, I sometimes had to go back two months earlier.

Going to the doctor's was like listening to a broken record. I'd tell them I'm in pain and they'd basically say, "No you're not." I guess they really don't believe us when we tell them our backs or our hips hurt because the standard response seems to be, "There's no pain with scoliosis."

Instead, they turn it around and ask psychological questions: "How's everything going at home?" "Are you having problems with any friends?" "How are your grades?" "Do you struggle in any subjects?"

Like an obedient patient, I answered everything appropriately, but felt like this was the doctor's way of blaming my pain on something other than the scoliosis. What always confused me was why would I lie to the very people who were supposed to be helping me? It felt like my doctors didn't believe that my pain was real. Didn't they know how horrible that made me feel?

Mom: If Rachel wasn't complaining of so much back pain, I would have never looked at her back and seen how significant her scoliosis had progressed. Doesn't that tell you something? No one was ever able to answer this question.

Rachel: Needless to say, nothing ever came from these earlier visits. At times, I think my doctor actually felt bad that she couldn't explain why my back hurt so much.

Mom: Our orthopedist recommended that Rachel begin two or three days of physical therapy each week to strengthen muscles that were being weakened from bracing. She also wanted Rachel to be treated once a week by a particular therapist who would concentrate on muscle strengthening for children afflicted by scoliosis.

EVERYTHING HAPPENS FOR A REASON

Rachel: On the very first appointment with the physical therapist, she pointed out the parts of my body that were being weakened from the scoliosis. I have to admit, I was surprised how hard it was to do the simplest exercises. Since I was still suffering with pain primarily located in my mid and upper back, the therapist tried to work the problem area out with an aggressive massage.

Mom: Once again, Rachel did not seem to benefit from this particular therapist's method for relieving her pain. As nice as she was, Rachel was still in pain. I needed to find another alternative for treatment.

Rachel: I couldn't move; her hands were pressing very hard on certain areas of my back. I later learned that she was trying to release one of the many trigger points (muscle spasms) that I had all over my upper back. I knew after that session that I was through for a while with people trying to help me with my pain.

Mom: Ironically, it was at the end of this session when the therapist mentioned that there was another girl in the waiting area who also had scoliosis, and was starting a support group for kids. "Would you be interested in meeting her?"

Rachel: Up to that point, I never met anyone else with scoliosis. She handed me a flyer and told me about a support group she wanted to begin, and asked if I would be interested in going. I eagerly said "yes" and in turn I gave her my telephone number.

Rachel: People often tell me I'm an old soul. I think one of the reasons they tell me that is because I think much deeper than most kids my age. For example, if I never went to this therapist, I would have never met Leah Stoltz, a young girl who would later become an important part of my life.

Mom: When I first met Leah, I was immediately impressed with how well she spoke. For being only thirteen, she was very mature. I was quickly drawn to her warm smile and courageous outlook regarding her condition. Already braced two years, for twenty-two hours a day, I listened in awe as she handed us a flyer announcing the start of her own support group for girls with scoliosis. It was her intention to share whatever she learned and then talk openly about the everyday challenges of bracing. Impressed with her positive attitude, I left optimistic that this group might be exactly what Rachel needed.

Several days later, Leah's mom, Robin, called. We talked for a while and I felt an instant connection with her. Now more than ever, I was truly getting excited about this support group. Before we ended our conversation, we mutually chose the date and the place of the first meeting. On Sunday, August 6, 2006, Rachel and I, along with three other moms and their daughters, arrived at their home.

I'M NOT ALONE

Rachel: Before the summer ended, I attended my first support group meeting at Leah's home. Scared at first, my nerves quickly disappeared as Leah began to talk to us about issues that affected her most when she was first braced, like clothing.

"Has this ever happened to you?" Leah asked as she held up a DKNY shirt. "You have your favorite shirt on over your brace and there are holes."

I remembered nodding my head and thinking to myself, "I'm not alone." Someone was verbally expressing the frustrations of wearing something you really like, maybe only once, and then having it ruined by something you hated … your brace.

As Leah continued to talk, she explained the importance of layering. She gave us tips on how to layer our clothes so the straps on our braces wouldn't be seen. I soon nicknamed her the "Queen of Layering." Leah's valuable tips on layering the clothes with a tank top on underneath to cover the bulkiness helped prevent the outer shirt from getting damaged. Leah also knew something about sleeping more comfortably at night. She suggested putting a pillow under our legs to balance the unevenness the brace put us in while lying down.

"Doing this little trick," Leah said, "will help you sleep more comfortably at night."

By the end of our first meeting I was blown away with everything I had just learned. On the way home, I went clothes shopping with my mom and actually had fun. That evening when I had to go to bed, I slept great. Do you want to know why? Because I slept with a pillow under my legs! Needless to say I was very anxious to return the following month to learn more of Leah's "scoliosis survival skills."

Mom: As the girls walked off to talk privately about their issues, the moms began to bond about doctors, back braces, and the overwhelming frustrations of whether or not we were making the right decisions for our girls. By the end of our first meeting, both Rachel and I left their home smiling and feeling like a weight was just lifted from our shoulders. Who would have ever thought that talking to strangers would have been so effective?

Rachel: Somehow each month, Leah knew what we needed to talk about. One month we might discuss our innermost feelings of wearing the brace, how and why we felt the brace changed us, the anxieties we had right before our next doctor's appointment, or the fears someone might be going through anticipating having corrective surgery. Other times we'd talk about the different obstacles we faced being teenage girls, like problems in school or the dreaded girl drama.

> One of the things that made me so proud to be part of this group was that there were no clicks, no popular girls, no mean girls, just girls with scoliosis whose goal was to help each other.

Leah, being the oldest, was a great role model; she always knew what to say. I remember once telling her, and the group, that I was having problems with some girls in school. Her genuine concern for my situation meant so much to me. It wasn't so much what she said, (though it did help) but how she reacted and listened. No matter the topic of conversation, the bottom line was that we supported each other and developed our very own "scoli-family."

The bond we all made is hard to explain, but we knew we wanted to continue to reach out and help others. Eventually, we decided to name our support group the "Curvy Girls."

Who would have imagined a random meeting in a physical therapist's office would have led to this?

Mom: As the first year passed, Rachel continued to be closely monitored. At each follow-up appointment, we would learn if her curve progressed, if her Risser score went up, and if she grew any taller. Taking new x-rays every four months was something I hated putting Rachel through, but we had no choice. During this time, as Rachel grew, her curve basically remained the same. It would go up 2° and then back down 2°. I attributed this success to Rachel's strict discipline on complying with her bracing. Never did I see her trying to cheat or even loosen her straps during those years.

Rachel: When I finally got my period, I was so excited. Most girls probably wouldn't have cared so much, but for a girl who has scoliosis, getting your period means that an end to bracing is finally in sight. In the next eighteen months to two years after beginning menstruating, the spine will stop growing and then we can finally be brace-free. However, it was during this time that a few of the girls in our support group, who were braced longer than I, found out they had to have surgery. This was a difficult time for me as I watched these girls, who I now considered my friends, prepare for surgery. I couldn't help but begin to wonder, "Am I wearing my brace for no reason? Will I end up having surgery just like them?"

Mom: I was surprised to hear Rachel question whether or not bracing was really worth it. I felt like I needed to discuss this further with her, fearing that she might begin to give up as well. I explained to Rachel that if these girls never wore their brace, their curves would have probably progressed to even a higher degree. Plus, the sad reality is that some kids might progress to the point of surgery regardless how much they braced. No one knows for sure. All I do know is that giving up the brace is not the smartest decision, especially when we know the brace is working for you.

Rachel later learned that some of the girls admitted to having stopped wearing their brace consistently. They encouraged the other girls not to make the same mistake. On a positive note, within eight months of her period, Rachel's pelvic growth plate (Risser) went from a 1 to a 4-5, which meant her growing was really coming to an end. I was so excited to share this great news with family and friends who were our anchors during this time.

REGAINING CONTROL

Rachel: By the end of the sixth grade, I was having a hard time bracing everyday in school. On top of it being difficult to wear, I was dealing with insensitive teachers. Sitting or standing for long periods was very uncomfortable, and while not often, sometimes I needed to walk around or go to the nurse just to take a little break from the brace. I actually had a teacher make fun of me when I asked to go to the nurse twice in one week.

Not only was I embarrassed by his rude comments, now I was more determined than ever to find another solution for not bracing during school hours. Oh, and P.S., in case you were wondering, my mom took care of that problem when she confronted the teacher on his insensitivity.

After this experience, my mom agreed to let me change my bracing hours. I think she finally began to understand what I was going through on a daily basis. I would now wear my brace from 3:00 p.m. to 7:00 a.m., and I felt like I could deal with the restrictions better at home than in school. Teachers and classmates never fully understood how hard it was to wear this turtle shell corset under my clothes.

A simple thing like dropping your pen, paper, or book, which would take anyone only a second to retrieve, is a project for someone strapped in this medieval harness offering no flexibility.

Not wearing the brace to school was the best decision I think we ever made. I actually felt happier. I never had to be reminded to put the brace on or to be checked to see if it was put on tight enough. Would you believe that I actually didn't mind wearing the brace anymore? It was true. I actually felt better in the brace than I did out of it. It's amazing how much easier bracing became once I took back some control in my life.

Mom: Sadly, Rachel's back pain continued, and though I tried everything from physical therapy to chiropractic treatments, the only thing that actually gave her any relief was massage therapy. While continuing our monthly support group meetings, I soon learned there were many other girls who also suffered with back pain. It will always confuse me why doctors insist there is no pain associated with this disease.

SEPTEMBER 15th

Rachel: It seemed like the typical routine appointment. Each visit started out the same, x-rays and then waiting. This time however, I was feeling a little more nervous than usual for the x-ray results because I had a secret that I had kept to myself.

"Mom, I'm afraid I might have screwed everything up. I've slacked off an hour or two several times over the last couple of weeks, and now I'm worried that my curve might have gotten worse!" I quickly blurted out.

Jokingly, my mom remarked, "What is this, confession time? Relax. You've been so good. A few hours shouldn't have made that much of a difference." Having my mom say that did help, but I wasn't stupid. The x-ray results are the only thing I could go by.

"You're brace-free!" said the physician assistant as she opened the door.

I was completely stunned by the words that came out of her mouth.

"Go ahead, get dressed. I'll give you a moment, and then we'll talk," were her exact words, and then she gently closed the door.

My jaw dropped. I looked over at my mom as she rushed over to hug me and we instantly began to cry.

"It's over, Rachel. You did it," my mom whispered in my ear as the tears began to fall. When the physician assistant returned, she opened the door and saw us crying.

"What's with the crying? This is happy news!"

Still crying, I managed to say, "You don't understand how hard this was for me, and now you're telling me it's over. It doesn't seem real."

She smiled and said, "You can put a girl in a brace and she'll cry, take her out and she'll still cry!"

Mom: Rachel beat the odds. From the first day we were told she needed to be braced, we were forewarned that there was a strong likelihood she would end up needing corrective spine surgery. Ironically, she had everything going against her. She was an eleven year old with a zero Risser, and a 35° curve that meant a lot of growing was still ahead of her. Our only option was to brace her and monitor her growth. Needless to say, this process of "wait-and-see" left us all very anxious and frightened. And yet we did it. No, I stand corrected, Rachel did it; she beat the odds!

Today, when I reflect over these past few years on everything she has gone through, I'm overwhelmed with pride. I cannot adequately express how amazed I am by the strength that she found within herself at such a young age.

A few years ago, Rachel let me read a journal entry she had written in the sixth grade. The theme was, "If you had a chance to change one thing about yourself, what would it be?" Though most children her age would have written, "Not to have scoliosis" or "Not to have to wear a back brace," Rachel chose "nothing," and explained why. She wrote, "We all have obstacles in our life we're meant to overcome, and dealing with scoliosis must be mine." Rachel concluded that if she wished her scoliosis away, it would have been like wishing a part of her didn't exist.

I WOULDN'T CHANGE A THING

Rachel: I couldn't believe that my journey had ended. No more holes in my shirt, no more awkward sleeping positions, no more back brace! I walked out of that office happier than I could have ever thought imaginable. Once in the car, my mom and I joked that I just got a belated birthday gift, since my birthday had just passed on September 1st. Before we left the parking lot, my mom began calling everyone in the family to tell them that I was brace-free. I, unfortunately, couldn't stop crying, but continued to repeat the words, "I'm free; I'm really free." The reality that it was truly over took a while for me to process.

There's no doubt in my mind that I could not have accomplished two and a half years of bracing without the support from my family and the Curvy Girls. Having scoliosis made me grow up a lot faster than other kids my age. Coping with the drama in middle school and high school is difficult enough, but when you add scoliosis and bracing into the mix, it's overwhelming.

If you are reading my story right now, and you're depressed and suffering with your brace, don't start hating life because of this condition. Please learn from the mistakes we made through my bracing. Remember bracing isn't comfortable, but it is bearable. If you're in pain with your brace, speak up. Allow our personal journeys to give you the confidence that we once lacked.

The diagnosis of this disease first changed me for the worst, and then inspired me to become a better person. If given the opportunity to change my past, I wouldn't change a thing.

ALYSSA

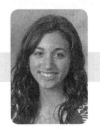

Age: 16

Braced at age 13

I like playing the viola. My friends are a huge part of my life, and I enjoy hanging out with them. I enjoy ice-skating and dancing. I love tap and jazz, and I skate three times a week.

Curvy Girls means so much to me. It has really helped me get through everything.

Alyssa's Message: Locate a Curvy Girls support group and attend their meetings. They will help you more than you'll ever know.

They Knew Best

Alyssa

I am sixteen years old and currently a junior in high school. I enjoy figure skating, dancing, and spending time with family and friends. I was diagnosed with scoliosis when I was twelve years old. At the time, I didn't know much about scoliosis. All I knew was that either my pediatrician or school nurse would check my back each year. The degree of curvature when I was first diagnosed was minimal, only 12°. My doctor said that my family and I should not be overly concerned because scoliosis was very common, especially in girls. I should, however, come back regularly just as a precaution. My mom recalled that this was the same protocol used when she had been diagnosed with scoliosis as a young teenager.

About a year passed and my curve hadn't changed much. It wasn't until the summer before eighth grade that my curve had gone to 17°, high enough to be put in a brace. I remember it like it was yesterday—the day my doctor told me I needed to be braced. I was to wear it for sixteen hours each day. He proceeded to show me what the brace would look like. It was a big, bulky, plastic object that definitely did not look comfortable at all. I thought that this man was crazy. He couldn't honestly think I would do this, even though I knew that I had to.

I couldn't believe this was happening to me. I tried not to let it affect me too much. I kept thinking that I still had time. After all, they had to measure me and then make the brace before I would even have to wear it.

I remembered the car ride home. I was sitting in the back seat, thinking about everything the doctor had just told me. It had all happened so quickly. Everything would change once I started wearing the brace. I knew this, and I couldn't keep back the tears.

"Why did this have to happen to me?" I said over and over again in my head. There was nothing I could do to change the situation, so I tried not to think about it too much.

49

Then came the day I received my first brace. I remember trying it on for the first time to make sure it fit. The doctor told me to sit down and see how it felt. It was so hard to sit! My back was completely straight. It felt so weird to be in this position. However, the brace fit fine. It would just take some getting used to.

The first night wearing the brace was a nightmare. There was a lot of pain in my back because my spine was being moved in a way that it never had before. The brace was extremely uncomfortable and was digging into my sides really hard. After hours of trying to endure the pain, I eventually gave up. It was already one o'clock in the morning and I was done trying to sleep with it. The brace was so painful, digging into my skin, that I developed a huge bruise. My mom and I took several trips to the orthotist for adjustments. More padding was added onto the back and side. The brace did get more and more comfortable to sleep in and within a month it was no trouble at all.

Though I got used to the brace, I most certainly did not find it easy to always maintain the required hours. Because I spent early morning and late afternoon hours out of my brace for activities like ice-skating, I had to wear my back brace during all school hours.

If I didn't have an after-school activity, I was able to keep it off for school. These were my favorite days because I didn't have to worry about taking it off during gym, or not being able to pick up pencils for other kids when they dropped them. You may laugh, but this happens very often! Another great thing about not having to wear the brace to school was that I was able to wear whatever clothes I wanted without having to worry about hiding my brace. To say that this was not a difficult feat to overcome would be a complete and utter lie. In fact, it was anything but easy. As much as I tried to make it work, it wasn't working. I didn't want anybody looking at me differently because I wore a brace.

All I wanted was to fit in and
be "normal" like everyone else.

Only my very close friends knew about it and I even had a hard time telling them. All of this changed about a year after I had been religiously wearing the brace.

At the beginning of that summer, my parents found an article in the daily newspaper about a girl nearby who had started a scoliosis group. She was only a year older than me, so my parents thought it would be a great opportunity for me to talk to other girls my age who were going through the exact same thing as I was. However, I *refused* to go. The last thing I wanted was to talk to other people about this. Fortunately for me, my parents weren't going to let me get away with not going. I remember quite clearly how my dad had to practically drag me into the car as I was screaming that I didn't want to go. While I might not have been all that thrilled at the time, today I am very thankful that my parents did this for me. I joined the group the summer going into ninth grade and stayed ever since.

The Curvy Girls means so much to me because it has helped me in many ways. In the beginning I was always self-conscious about wearing my brace and afraid of telling my friends. Then, I joined the Curvy Girls. While I had a lot of support from my friends and family, being able to talk about it with people my age is exactly what I needed to do. It made me realize that there are other people going through the same thing and that it isn't as bad as you think. We all have our own personal challenges and insecurities to face and scoliosis just happens to be mine. As time went on, I soon began to notice that I was able to open up more to my friends. I was still shy, but it was a big step in the right direction for me to let go of my secret.

I wore the brace for sixteen hours a day for two years, up until November of my sophomore year of high school. As much as I hated the brace, I wore it because I hoped that, in the end, it would pay off. Thankfully, it did. Now I only wear my brace at night.

If you have a positive attitude towards bracing, and you don't worry about what other people may think, you will feel so much better. I always used to feel like I was hiding something, and I hated that. It really helped to be able to talk to the girls in the group who were having the same problems with the brace as I did. Having them share their advice and experiences was invaluable to me. Thanks to the Curvy Girls, my outlook on scoliosis and the importance of wearing the brace has changed.

Since my journey is almost over, I plan on continuing to help the newer members of the group, as I was helped when I first joined. As difficult as these past years have been, I got through it because I had the support of my family, friends and the Curvy Girls. I believe my experiences have molded me into a stronger person, and for that I am very grateful.

Nothing Like Mine

Jeanne

When my daughter was first diagnosed with scoliosis, just shy of her twelfth birthday, I wasn't very alarmed. After all, I was diagnosed with scoliosis as a young teen and I never had any problems. I knew that scoliosis in girls is fairly common. What I didn't know, however, was that my daughter's scoliosis would be very different from mine.

Initially, my daughter was screened with an x-ray every four months. The first year, there were no changes in her spinal curve, just as I had suspected would happen. It wasn't until the second year of surveillance that I realized her scoliosis was quite different. Her curve increased enough to warrant being placed in a scoliosis brace for sixteen hours a day. In the beginning it was so hard for Alyssa to fall asleep wearing the brace. I'll never forget the sleepless nights and tears for both my daughter and myself. Eventually, she did get comfortable and we slept once again.

My daughter was a brave young girl, rarely complaining about having to wear her brace. That is not to say things always went smoothly. At times, she struggled. There were days when she couldn't find the mental strength to wear her brace to school, so on those days she didn't wear it. Luckily, she didn't have too many of those days.

I recall countless visits to the orthotist's office for adjustments to be made on a new brace. During these times a new brace meant bruises, rashes, and downright pain until they made the necessary adjustments for it to fit properly. We always dreaded the necessity for a new brace, but eventually it always worked out.

I believe my daughter's biggest obstacle with scoliosis was trying to overcome her need to hide her brace from her friends. This caused her much stress and worry. She worried about her brace being noticeable under her clothing. She didn't want her teachers or her friends to know she wore a brace. She didn't want to be treated differently.

This is where the support group for girls with scoliosis helped her immensely. Initially, she was not interested in attending a Curvy Girls support group. It meant having to talk about something she did not want to talk about. We tried in vain to convince her that a support group would have a positive effect on her, however, she didn't want to hear it. We all but carried her to her first meeting.

Today she attends of her own free will and desire. That first step was extremely difficult, until she realized how helpful it is to talk to other young people who are living with scoliosis. I cannot stress enough the importance of finding a support group. It made a world of difference to my daughter.

Recently, Alyssa received very good news from her doctor. At the age of fifteen, she has reduced her brace time to only wearing it to sleep. She is literally counting the days with a calendar at her bedside, marking off each and every month that will bring her closer to the moment she will be brace-free.

The hope is that she will only have to wear the brace for one more year, and finally be able to say goodbye to her brace, along with the concern of ever needing corrective scoliosis surgery.

ESTHER

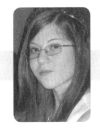

Age: 16

Braced at age 9; Spinal Fusion at age 14–upper thoracic curve

Continues to be braced for lumbar curve

I enjoy playing the piano and I'm active in student government as class treasurer. I love theater and chorus. Curvy Girls helped me feel more confident in myself and know I am not alone.

Esther's Message: Talking to other kids who have been through the same experiences makes everything so much easier.

The Big Event

Esther and Sheryl

Mom: When an athlete trains for the big race, they train hard. It is all about getting your mind, body, and spirit ready. Everything has to be focused for the big event. But who helps prepare your child and family for surgery?

As a family, we had lots of practice for surgery. They say practice makes it easier. If you've been around the course before, you know how to finish the race. You know what to expect. Spinal surgery was to be Esther's sixth surgery. Esther has a syndrome called Cardio-Facial-Syndrome. She is missing part of her 22nd chromosome and was diagnosed while in the neonatal intensive care unit, when she was born five weeks early. Esther has undergone two cardiac surgeries, one tonsillectomy, and two surgeries on her palate. Her last surgery was done when she was six years old. We believed we were finished, and then seven years later we had to get ready for another surgery.

Esther: I don't remember any of the surgeries except the one when I was six years old. My mom stayed with me, and I was only in the hospital for two days. I remember getting lots of gifts, and having to eat soft foods after surgery. My biggest issue about my spine surgery was that my Bat Mitzvah was scheduled for the same time I was going to have surgery, and I didn't want to cancel my Bat Mitzvah. We had planned a great trip to Israel, and I couldn't believe this was happening.

Mom: As parents, we were anticipating the need for spinal surgery at some time. But we had always thought it would be later, or hoped it would not be at all. Esther was, and is still, very small for her age. At fourteen years old, she was 4 feet 5 inches tall. We had hoped she would not need surgery until she had stopped growing, maybe at sixteen. But at thirteen, she started to go through puberty, and then her spine progressed from 35° to 60° in a very short period of time.

We had planned her Bat Mitzvah trip one year before, never thinking we might have to be making a choice between surgery and her trip to Israel. Most kids have their surgery during the summer or vacation time, so they won't have to miss too much school. As a family we made the decision to do both, go to Israel in the beginning of the summer and then have the surgery toward the end, missing only the first month of school. Esther was a good student and we had confidence she could make up the work.

Esther: I have been wearing a brace since I was nine years old. I had to wear my brace for twenty-three hours a day. I had hoped that surgery meant I would be rid of my brace, but unfortunately it did not work out that way. I have an "S" curve and my surgery was going to correct my upper spine. The doctors hoped the surgery would help my lower curve as well.

I was hoping to throw out my old clothes and go shopping. My brace before surgery had a shoulder strap that was difficult to hide. My clothes were always two sizes bigger in order to hide the brace.

> I was dreaming of the day
> I could wear normal clothes,
> tight clothes that could show off my curves.

Mom: So our plans were made for surgery and our trip to Israel. When our spine doctor told us we could not delay the surgery any longer, we had another surprise. He informed us that he would not be doing the surgery, but would refer us to a colleague who would do the surgery for Esther. Esther always has challenging surgeries; nothing is ever easy. Her surgeries are always difficult and we appreciated our doctor's assessment and judgment. He had our daughter's best interest in mind. He is a fine surgeon and physician, so referring Esther was the right thing to do for her. When she had her second heart surgery, it was complicated. Most kids who have septal defects have one or two holes in the ventricle wall, Esther had what they call "Swiss cheese." She had several large holes and hundreds of small holes, and there were not many surgeons who could do her surgery.

Dr. Oheneba Boachie-Adjei at Hospital for Special Surgery in New York was someone who we were very familiar with. I had heard about his reputation for several years, and had decided that if Esther ever needed surgery, he was the man to do it. He had the skills to do the difficult cases. So we felt confident Esther was going to the right place, with the right surgeon.

Esther: My parents' confidence in the surgeon, made me feel confident too. I knew my parents did a lot of research to find the best doctor. Though my surgeries, I am told, have been difficult, they always turn out well. I have come a long way. I have survived, and lived, when some were not sure I would. I am living proof that anything is possible.

On the radio and TV there were lots of advertisements about the hospital we were going to. It was named the "Best Orthopedic Hospital" with the "Best Nursing Care." I was scared about what was going to happen to me, but I felt confident that I was going to be all right.

Mom: Having the right mindset that you are in the best place is important. As a nurse, I know there are many good places for surgery, many good doctors. But it helps to have the confidence that you are in the best place for your child.

Before our trip to Israel, Esther had to undergo pre-surgical testing. It is routine, but in Esther's case, nothing is routine. My husband, Marty, took her for the appointment. We live in the suburbs and they had to take the train to get to Manhattan. An important pre-surgical assessment is seeing the pulmonologist and having pulmonary function tests prior to surgery. Children with severe upper curves have some degree of pulmonary compromise before surgery. This is usually the reason for surgery because the spine is starting to affect the internal organs. When my husband came home from the pre-surgical visit, I did not expect the news he was going to share. Marty told me that Esther had failed her pulmonary function tests badly. Her lungs were compromised. In order to give her lungs a chance to re-expand, they recommended she be on a ventilator for three days after surgery. Everything changed with that news.

I had not paid attention to signs that Esther was having breathing trouble. When Esther came home telling me she couldn't run the mile in school because her chest hurt so much that she was crying, I just thought it was because she never ran a mile before. After all, Esther had never been an athlete and didn't do sports. I felt so bad that I hadn't taken her words seriously.

Pulmonary function tests should be done for kids with scoliosis who have significant upper curves. I had spoken to other people who had the surgery, but no one had been on a ventilator after surgery. As a nurse, I know we do this surgery in my hospital and it is not the routine procedure that requires someone to be on a ventilator afterwards. But Esther's surgeries are never the routine, and this was proving to be the case again. Esther had been on a ventilator after surgery when she had her heart surgeries, but that was more common for those procedures. That was different. This was going to be challenging for my husband and me, and especially for Esther.

Esther: My parents never told me I was going to be on a ventilator after surgery. I would have probably been more scared than I already was. But they did tell me I was going to have a tube in my mouth and I might not be able to speak for a day or two after surgery. So my mom and I talked about how we would communicate if I couldn't talk. We would use hand signals. I could give thumbs up if I was okay or thumbs down if I needed something or if something was not right. We had a routine of telling each other that we loved one another with hand signals. I would point to myself for "I." I would hug myself for "love," and would point to my mom or dad for "you." Telling each other, "I love you," reminds you that we are there for each other. It makes you feel safe.

Mom: Our trip to Israel was everything we could have imagined and more. Her Bat Mitzvah was at the Masada. It was over 100° F. We took off the brace during the ceremony; otherwise, she might have fainted from heat exhaustion. As wonderful as the trip was, there was always the thought that when we returned home, surgery was waiting.

Her Bat Mitzvah reminded me of all she had gone through throughout her life, and what a great girl she had turned out to be. When she was an infant, she was very ill. There were times I was not sure she was going to make it. It was hard to imagine Esther at her Bat Mitzvah, singing her Hebrew so well and accomplishing much more than we ever could dream.

My method to deal with crisis is to cry. I am a big crybaby. Everyone who knows me, knows I cry. I rarely get through movies, weddings, or events without crying. Esther has seen me cry a million times, but sometimes it affects her.

Esther: At my Bat Mitzvah, my mom cried. In fact, the camera went directly to her, and we have the proof. She cries when she is happy, and when she is sad. She cries in the doctor's office, and sometimes it scares me when I don't understand why she is crying.

Mom: Israel helped us all spiritually. It put us in a good state of readiness. Prayers help. We all put a note in the Wailing Wall. It is a tradition to make a prayer, write it down, and put the note into the cracks in the wall. My note was that Esther was going to be all right. I have lots of friends and relatives who attend synagogue and church, so I asked everyone to pray for Esther's recovery. When we came home, we were as emotionally and spiritually ready as we could be.

Esther: The weeks before my surgery were all about getting ready for the day. I got new pajamas. I picked out new DVDs that I would watch after surgery. I started to pack and prepare. Presents started to arrive from my family and friends. I love presents! It felt like a celebration like a birthday, rather than going to surgery.

A few months before my surgery, I had seen a news article about a support group for scoliosis. My mom and I thought it would be great to talk to someone who had already had the surgery. We found the article on the Internet, and then identified two girls that had the surgery, Leah and Dominique. My mom talked to Leah's mom and then I spoke to Leah. Leah had her surgery a few weeks before and was doing really well. I asked her about the pain after surgery, and she said the medicine worked. She told me about the PCA (pain medicine pump) and how it helped with the pain.

After talking to Leah, I felt much better. I felt confident that if she was doing well, that I would be fine too. Then we called Dominique, who had surgery with the same surgeon that I was going to use. She was also doing very well. Talking to kids who have gone through what you are going to go through helps a lot. We had already missed that month's support group meeting, but I was going to try to attend the next meeting after my surgery.

Mom: Speaking to Robin, Leah, and Dominique made a world of difference to us. Esther was in the right frame of mind for surgery. Other girls did well, and so would my Esther. None of the girls had to undergo being on a ventilator. But we had made it through other challenges, and we would make it through this one. I had to pack for both Esther and myself since I was going to stay with Esther for the week. It is important to bring comfortable clothes and comfortable shoes. If you are planning to sleep in the hospital, plan on sleeping in the clothes you are wearing, and changing each day. The clothes you put on in the morning are the clothes for the day. We found out before we went to the hospital that there are showers for parents. Most pediatric hospitals have areas for parents to clean up, or at least a bathroom. Bring supplies to refresh yourself, because smelling is not an option.

> While your child is in the hospital,
> be sure to bring something to
> pass the time, and to keep your sanity.

For some it may mean reading, but for me, reading was not an option. While I love reading, I knew I could not concentrate. I needed some kind of mindless craft. The night before surgery, I dug out a sewing project that I had started ten years ago. It was a needlepoint kit that I knew I could work on, and it would provide me with a mindless project to do during the day and night while I was at Esther's bedside.

Esther: My mom arranged one more activity, which was to meet a nurse who would be at my surgery. My mom works at a hospital. After talking to another nurse, she told me that there was a nurse where my mom works who also works with my surgeon two days a week. My mom met her and she said she would be happy to meet with me. I asked her about the surgery. She told me I had the best surgeon, and she would meet me before surgery. I asked her how I would recognize her in the operating room with everyone wearing masks. She asked me, what my favorite color was, and I said, "Pink." She told me that she would be wearing a pink hat.

On the day before surgery, we slept at my uncle's apartment in New York City. We had to be at the hospital by 5:00 a.m. So sleeping close by meant we could get up by 4:00 a.m. and not have to travel from the suburbs. I was ready to get my surgery done and over. I was glad when the day came.

Just before the surgery, I saw my nurse. She was wearing a pink cap. I saw my doctor; he was ready. My parents were there. We took some pictures of my dad and I dressed for surgery. My dad was going to go with me to the operating room. I was ready and then my mom started to cry. We were ready, I was ready, and this was no time to be scared. We were in the best hospital, with the best surgeon, and I knew I was going to be just fine. I turned to my mom, and told her to, "SUCK IT UP."

And she did.

Mom: My tears immediately stopped when I heard those words. Everything went dry. We had done our job to prepare our child. She was ready. She was confident; this was not the time to show weakness. This was not the time to show that I was afraid. I needed to show confidence, as she was showing the world she was the champion. She was brave enough for all of us. Somehow I did my part and got composure. The last words Esther heard before she went into the operating room were that we loved her and we would be right by her side when the surgery was over.

Once she left, I had my cry. While we waited, I got ready for her road to recovery. Seeing her after surgery was going to be tough. We still had to face Esther being on a ventilator, and I was not sure how she would react. As a nurse, I knew she would be medicated so she would not fight the machine.

After surgery, they let us see her in the recovery room. She was on the ventilator and was doing well. The doctor told us the surgery went well. She was awake when we approached her bedside. She looked at me, gave me the thumbs up and did her hand signal to tell us she loved us. I knew her mind was fine and that her body would recover. I cried, but it was a good cry. We were on our road to getting better.

Esther: It's hard to remember my recovery in the hospital. Maybe it's from the anesthesia or the pain medicine but I have no memory of any pain or being on a ventilator. What I do remember is talking to other girls who went through the same thing. Soon after my surgery I went to my first Curvy Girls meeting and finally got to meet Dominique and Leah. I think what I learned the most through this experience is that having someone to speak to before and after surgery is key. The Curvy Girls gave me confidence, allowing me to give back, helping others as Leah helped me.

DANIELLE

Age: 17

Braced at age 14

I have been dancing for years. I also play tennis and like to go skiing. I play the violin and enjoy reading.

The Curvy Girls was a way for me to receive advice and support while I was wearing my brace, and now it is a way for me to give back and help other girls who are going through similar situations.

Danielle's Message: Who said that feeling different has to make you feel bad about yourself? Scoliosis made me different in a way that I am proud of.

Staying Above the Curve

Danielle

"Danielle? The doctor's ready to see you now. You can follow me." I followed the nurse to the small room in which I had been so many times. I was used to this by now, for I had been doing it for quite a few years.

"The doctor will see you in a few minutes," she said, "but first you can follow me so we can take some x-rays."

I walked behind her down the hallway where I had followed her so many times. It was a standard routine for me. I didn't think anything would be different this time, but I was wrong.

YOUNG AND NAÏVE

It all started when I was in sixth grade. I was at my pediatrician's office for my annual check-up. Everything was going well and it seemed that I was perfectly healthy. Then, my doctor asked me to bend over so he could check my back. I did as I was told and, after a few seconds, he told me to stand up. Next, I heard some news that I wasn't expecting at all. He told me that I had scoliosis, but that it was very slight. I only had a curve of about 12°. Although my curve was subtle, my doctor recommended that I see an orthopedist so my curve could be monitored. Even though I was somewhat shocked to hear this news, I thought nothing of it. I was still young and I didn't think that it would ever affect me in a negative way. Little did I know that by the time freshman year of high school arrived, it would be one of the hardest and most challenging years of my life.

For the next few years, my life went on normally. I did everything that normal kids did. I played sports, danced, and hung out with friends. My scoliosis didn't bother me at all. I didn't feel any different from the kids at school. No one noticed that I was different because, in truth, I really wasn't. However, my curve had not stopped progressing.

65

BEING BRACED

I went to the orthopedist every six months. Each time he would take x-rays, he informed me and my parents that my curve had progressed. During one visit in June, I went to the orthopedist as usual. He took some x-rays and then I waited in the familiar, tiny room for my results. Even though I didn't realize it at the time, the news he told my parents and I would soon change my life.

The doctor informed us that my curve had progressed six degrees, from 18° to 24°. He said that it was time to put me in a brace. He recommended that I see an orthotist so that I could have a brace made. This was the most shocking news I had ever heard, but I kept my composure. I had no idea what to expect about the brace. I did not know what it would look like or what it would feel like to wear. The orthopedist said that I had nothing to worry about, but I couldn't help but be nervous.

I had to go to the orthotist right away because I would be leaving for sleep away camp in a few days, and it would take time for the brace to be made. When I arrived at his office, I was extremely nervous. I had not the faintest idea of what he was going to do, but it didn't take long for me to find out. As soon as I met the orthotist, he made me feel at ease. He calmed me down, explained how he would measure me for a brace, and described what would be expected of me during the next year or so. He said that I would have to wear the brace for at least twenty-two hours a day in order for it to do its job, to hold my spine in place and prevent the curve from progressing. One thing that made me particularly happy was that I was allowed to be out of the brace to attend my dance classes. Dance is something I love to do—a time that I could enjoy and be free of my brace.

After a long discussion of what to expect of the brace, it was finally time to be measured. The orthotist asked me to stand as straight as possible, and he wrapped me up like a mummy in a plaster cast, which would later harden and form a mold of my body. I had to hold very still so that the cast could be made properly. After he removed the plaster, he told me that I should enjoy myself at sleep away camp and not worry about anything. This made me feel a lot better and, for a fleeting moment, the thought of having a scoliosis brace didn't seem so bad anymore. Little did I know what I was in for . . .

EVERYTHING CHANGES WITH A BRACE

The next few weeks went by rather quickly. Sleep away camp was fun, but I knew that when I got back, my life would be very different. I only had a month left before starting high school, and I wanted to adjust to the brace as much as I possibly could. Putting the brace on for the first time was not a fun experience. It was very constricting and hard to move in. It was also a little hard to breathe because it didn't allow my stomach to expand fully. Luckily, however, I had a month to adjust before school started.

Freshman year was nothing like I had ever imagined. I never thought that I would start my first day of high school wearing a scoliosis brace. One of the things I hated the most about the brace was that I couldn't wear what I wanted for fear that people would be able to see the brace through my clothes. I basically had to wear baggy sweatshirts everyday to hide the brace, which made me really upset. Only my close friends knew about the brace and I guess no one else noticed that I was wearing it. I also hated how I had to go to the nurse's office every other day to change in and out of the brace for gym. It was a big hassle, but I got through it because the nurses were extremely nice and understanding.

DIFFERENT AND PROUD

To help me get through this tough time, I also joined a scoliosis support group, which was started by another girl just like me. This group allowed me to connect and share my stories with other girls who had similar situations to mine. Not only did I feel supported in this group, but it also gave me the chance to give my support to other girls with scoliosis. Joining this group made me realize how lucky I was not to have needed back surgery. Many of the girls in the group who wore back braces still needed surgery when their curves progressed.

Wearing a scoliosis brace was the biggest challenge of my life so far. It made me change my view about life. Even though I had many days when I felt really depressed and upset about my situation, this whole experience made me realize how lucky I was not to have an even worse problem. It made me realize how many people there are in this world with severe disabilities that affect them every day of their lives. I wouldn't even call having scoliosis a disability, especially now that I don't have to wear the brace anymore. I am just like everyone else, yet having scoliosis makes me different in a way that I am proud of. I believe that every person in this world has at least one major challenge to get through in his or her lives, and I believe that this was mine.

This experience has made me a stronger person overall. I am ready to face new challenges whenever I need to, because I have been through the biggest one of all.

Would've, Could've, Should've...

Susan

I'm not worried. That was my reaction during Danielle's bend-over examination, when her pediatrician stated that the left side of her upper back was slightly higher than the right side. I could barely see it. He said it was nothing to worry about right now, but suggested that I take her to a specialist to have it checked.

We went to the orthopedist soon after that. I hadn't anticipated that we would be going every few months for x-rays and check-ups. Danielle was eleven going on twelve. My biggest worry at the time was repeated radiation from x-rays beginning at such a young age. We learned about scoliosis and how it could progress once a child hit a growth spurt. We learned about the degrees of curvature of the spine, and that Danielle would have to wear a brace or have surgery if her "number" reached a certain point. My main concern was still the x-rays. Perhaps because Danielle's curve was small, it did not occur to me to fret about the possibility of future treatment.

Danielle's curve increased slightly over the next two years, but she still didn't need a brace. Even though she looked like she was leaning to the left, neither of us was worried about it. It wasn't visible when she was wearing clothes. Then, at one of her checkups, we found that her curve had increased 6°. That was when we heard the words, "You have to wear a brace." I was shocked. Even though I had been informed about this as a possibility, I wasn't prepared for it. I felt even worse when Danielle started to cry. She was going to have to wear a brace for one and a half to two years, twenty-three hours a day.

Why hadn't I researched anything about scoliosis and braces? During the two years of monitoring her condition, why didn't it occur to me to look up any of this? I could have kicked myself. I didn't know what the brace would look or feel like, and I never thought to ask. Somehow I pictured it as a type of Victorian corset, and that Danielle would be able to move freely while wearing it.

The next shock was finding out that the brace would be hard plastic made from a mold of her body, with straps attached to close it so that it would fit snugly. The orthotist put Danielle at ease about the entire process, and we left his office with the feeling that everything would work out. She had a month to adjust to the brace before starting high school. I went to the library and read some books about scoliosis. I gave some to Danielle to read. For me, it would be all right as long as Danielle was all right. At that point, it seemed like she was in a positive frame of mind and would be able to manage this period in her life with little angst. I offered her words of encouragement and truly believed that she could handle it.

Was it wishful thinking? I still wasn't too worried, until the reality of wearing a brace to a new school hit her like a ton of bricks. It was uncomfortable for her to sit down, and she couldn't wear form-fitting clothes over the brace, so she wore baggy sweatshirts to hide it. She hated that she couldn't wear the clothes she liked. She told only her close friends; she didn't want anyone else to know. She was mortified when a classmate asked her to pick up a pencil that had rolled next to her chair. She couldn't bend over to get it and had to kick it to him. I had no first-hand experience with any of this, so I couldn't tell her that I knew what she was going through. I tried to be sympathetic, but I felt helpless to help her. It felt terrible to not be able to soothe her. After all, isn't that part of a mother's job? She called me at work almost every day after school, sounding as though she were in great distress. One day, I dropped everything and rushed home. I needed to make sure she was all right.

Despite the initial emotional turmoil, Danielle and I survived her brace experience. My feelings mirrored her feelings. If she had a good day, I had a good day. Throughout the bracing period, I was worried mostly about preserving her sanity. I reassured her that she would get through this, but there were days when she didn't seem so sure. It was only after Danielle said that she needed a support group that I began to look for one. She wanted to meet kids her age who were going through the same thing. Even though she often said no one she knew had scoliosis, and that she felt alone in dealing with it, it never occurred to me that this was what she needed. I searched for a support group to help my daughter, not realizing that it would help me too.

DANIELLE

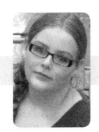

Age: 14

Spinal fusion surgery at age 13

I'm a fan of the Dallas Cowboys. I love cats, dogs and most animals. I also love playing the violin and listening to country music.

The Curvy Girls are loving, understanding, and my heroes.

Danielle's Message: Don't ever let any professional yell at you!

Getting It Straight
Danielle and Debbie

SHE HAS WHAT?

Mom: We were at the pediatrician's office for her yearly physical when the doctor had her bend down to touch her toes. The doctor was standing directly behind her and examining her back. I could tell something was wrong when the doctor's face suddenly became serious. Then I heard his bone chilling words, "Mom, look at this." I knew something was very wrong. I got up to observe what the doctor had seen—my daughter's curving spine.

My sweet little eleven-year-old child, who I always thought of as perfectly healthy, had a major defect. Aside from an ear infection, Danielle never had any health issues and yet, today, I'm being told that I need to make an appointment with a scoliosis orthopedic specialist.

Danielle: I have scoliosis.

You probably don't think scoliosis is so bad, right? Wrong. Scoliosis is the bending or curving of the spine, and when diagnosed early, bracing would be suggested to prevent your curve from progressing.

> Scoliosis normally is not physically
> life threatening, but psychologically,
> it's like a bomb destroying self-esteem
> and self-confidence in an instant.

ROUND 1

Mom: I kept telling Danielle not to jump to the worst-case scenario, "We will work through this together." When we arrived at our first orthopedic appointment, they took x-rays. Much to our shock, the doctor returned to report that Danielle needed surgery as soon as possible. Her curves were too severe to even be braced. We were told that if we did not take care of this, her vital organs could be affected.

Danielle: I had the worst feeling when I walked into the orthopedic exam room. I felt as if I was going to be told that I needed surgery. My mom assured me that I was dwelling on the negative. After two x-rays, I returned to the room. I sat down in the chair all hot and red-faced because of my fears. The doctor came in, pulled up the x-ray and said, "Well, you need surgery." Just like that. I not only had one curve, but I was lucky to have two. The top was 52° and the bottom was at 49°. No explaining, "This is like this because …" or "This is like that." I just shrugged it off because, as usual, I had prepared myself for the absolute worst.

Mom: Where do you get the strength to be strong so that your child doesn't see how out-of-your-mind scared you are? Where do you find the words to make her okay with the news she just received? I promised her we would try everything we could to fix it before we would even think about surgery, and I did. A friend of mine had a brother who was a chiropractor. While he was quite far from where we lived, we decided to make the trip twice a week. I was doing everything I could just to make this awful monster go away.

LET'S TRY A CHIROPRACTOR
Danielle: On the drive home it was all about scoliosis, scoliosis this, surgery that. "I was like, all right, I need surgery. Who cares?" Apparently, my mom does. A lot!

When we returned home, my mom began making phone calls. She conceived this great idea of taking me to a chiropractor. With his magical hands he was going to straighten my back out (or so we thought). His office was located in Huntington, New York, which was a little difficult because we lived forty-five minutes away. Meeting the chiropractor was a much better experience than meeting the orthopedist. He was very nice and understanding.

Mom: I appreciated how genuinely caring this chiropractor was to Danielle. He stretched her and gave exercises to help straighten her. Danielle's curves were significant. I could easily see that the top curve made one shoulder bulge out, causing her to lean to one side. The lower curve went in the opposite direction. He worked at adjusting her back and then measuring her legs to try and make them equal lengths.

My theory was to go steadily to the chiropractor in order to straighten her enough to be braced. We continued with this path for two months, and then I made an appointment for a second opinion with another spine specialist.

Danielle: There were no guarantees that the chiropractor could help, at least to the extent that my curve would decrease in order for a brace to help. It wasn't until later that I learned that being in a brace was no picnic either. Sometimes, I think I'm happier that I never had to go through years of bracing, if surgery was inevitable.

MEETING DR. RUDE

Mom: Our second consult was, sadly, very disappointing. This surgeon was nasty, with no bedside manner. After a few minutes of reviewing all of Danielle's x-rays, he began to berate me on what a terrible thing I'd been doing by trying to avoid surgery. The last words he spoke to us were, "She needs surgery. Just deal with it." Once again, I found myself having to be strong in order to guide my daughter through another terrible experience.

Danielle: I'm sitting in an orthopedic center, for another opinion. Minutes later, we meet this Dr. "Rude." My first impression of him was not the greatest, as I watched him drag his feet unwillingly into the exam room. He sat down and said, "So what's going on?" in a rather flat, blah voice. The expression on his face screamed, "Don't want to be here." We told him my story, and how we'd been working with a chiropractor. He immediately flipped out and started yelling at us. I guess that woke him because he went a little crazy. I started to get that heated feeling again. Sitting there about to explode, afraid to speak, I felt a part of me just shut down. I couldn't deal with what was being said. How does a doctor yell at a kid for having hope? Doesn't he know how wrong that is?

Mom: We returned to our chiropractor, believing that his treatment was at least keeping Danielle's body mobile. He had become a part of our life. I told him the story about our visit with our second opinion. Being a medical professional with warmth and compassion, he apologized for the other doctor's insensitive behavior. I asked him whom could I trust with Danielle's spine. He recommended Dr. Laurence Mermelstein of Long Island Spine Specialists. He told us that his mother-in-law was having surgery with him, and felt that he is one of the best. We made an appointment with Dr. Mermelstein for the following week.

I FINALLY HAD HOPE

Danielle: Ten days later, my mom was able to get an appointment with another orthopedist that came highly recommended. After we filled out a few papers, we waited only a couple of seconds and were called into an exam room to go over my medical history with one of the nurses. Now we waited for what seemed like hours. Finally the doctor came in. He listened to everything. He examined my spine and reviewed the digital x-rays with me; this is something no other ortho-pedic surgeon ever offered to do. I found this to be very helpful. At the end of the appointment, he told my mom and I what we suspected all along: I needed surgery. Bracing would not help me, since my curves were severe. By now, my top curve was 60° and the lower curve was 50°.

Mom: As we waited for this new doctor to come in, I couldn't help but reflect that this was now our third consultation. While trying to remain positive, in walks this young, friendly physician.

He looked at the x-rays we brought with us, and in a very calm voice said, "Well, Mom, you did everything you could do, now let me fix this. She will be as good as new." Danielle and I left this office feeling like a weight had been lifted. For the first time, I actually felt good about a surgeon.

Danielle: There was no doubt that I wanted Dr. Mermelstein to do my surgery. I not only liked him, but I felt comfortable with him, something I never experienced with the other surgeons we saw.

Before we left, I happened to notice flyers on the counter. The women behind the desk told us there would be a scoliosis walk in May and we should think about going. I wasn't overly interested, but my mom convinced me to go.

As we drove to Jones Beach on Long Island's South Shore, I couldn't help but notice the overcast sky and dark clouds. I half expected it to start pouring the minute we got there. Much to my surprise, it didn't. Shortly after we arrived, we started the walk.

MEETING THE CURVY GIRLS

Danielle: After walking for about a half mile, I spotted a pink shirt on one of the girls walking in front of me. I knew the pink shirts were being worn by girls who were either in a brace or had surgery. In other words, they were the Curvy Girls. And, of course, I didn't have the courage to talk to anyone. After walking about one mile, I saw Leah. People tried to convince me to go and talk with her. When I finally did, she was really sweet. Before the walk ended, I was invited to the next Curvy Girls meeting.

Mom: Danielle and I were excited to go to Leah's home. At first, Danielle was very quiet and shy, but I knew she would be okay. After Leah took the girls downstairs for their meeting, Robin, Leah's mom, began the parent meeting. She introduced me and asked me to share a little bit of what I'd been going through this past year. As strong as I thought I was, the reality that Danielle's surgery was only a week away was making me very emotional. I choked up as I shared all my fears with these perfect strangers. As odd as it might sound, I was never embarrassed. Every parent there understood my pain and fears. For people I just met, I knew instinctively that they genuinely cared about what I was going through. What more could I have asked for?

Danielle: When the girls and I went downstairs, I wasn't sure how comfortable I would be. Leah was going around the room getting updates on what was going on with everyone. When it was my turn, I was a bit shy, but I did open up. The more I spoke, the more comfortable I began to feel. I liked this group. I really liked them.

SURGERY DAY

Mom: The day of the surgery, I was so nervous. I had to make sure that I had everything for Danielle and myself because there was no way I would leave her. It was so hard when they wheeled her toward the operating room. The waiting took forever.

Danielle: The morning of my surgery, I woke up at some ridiculous hour, got dressed, and headed to Good Samaritan Hospital in West Islip with my family. My parents are divorced, so my dad met us there. I began to think how lousy it was that in a few hours I'd be having surgery. The reality started hitting me. I couldn't believe I had to go through this. Oh my God!

I was then moved to this room where people who are prepped for surgery have to wait. This is called "pre-op," where the nurses and physicians who do your surgery speak with you. Next, I was wheeled into the operating room. I kept thinking to myself, "This is not happening." Unfortunately, it was. The anesthesia put me to sleep, and the surgery was performed.

Mom: The surgery was about six hours start to finish. They finally came out to tell us that surgery was completed, and we would see her post-op in thirty minutes. We found out that her spine was worse than the x-rays showed. Apparently, her spine had progressed even in the past four months since the last x-rays. They inserted too many screws to remember, plus two titanium rods. She was fused from T4 to L4. Her top curve went from 60° plus to 20° and her bottom curve from 50° plus to 11°.

IT'S OVER

Danielle: I had no idea what time it was when I woke up. I knew I was in the recovery room, which in my hospital is the same as pre-op. There were nurses surrounding me, which seemed kind of scary. My throat was bone dry, so they gave me ice chips. My eyes and face were so swollen from laying face down for hours. I could hardly open my eyes. That was a good thing, because all I wanted to do was sleep. After a while, they let my parents in to see me in recovery. When they took me to my room in Pediatric Intensive Care, my parents followed.

Mom: I wish we had been given a word from the wise before we saw Danielle. No one warned us that her face would be four times its normal size due to lying face down for hours during surgery! Much to our relief, the next day it was almost back to normal.

Danielle: I slept most of the night and the next day. The following day, I heard someone was there to see me. It was Leah and her mom. They came to the hospital just to see me. They brought me a bag of goodies and got me a Mr. Strong pillow. They didn't forget me.

Mom: They kept Danielle sedated for the first couple of days. By the third day, they began weaning her off of the pain medicine, and got her up. That was a day I will never forget. She was screaming and upset and afraid all at once. The kind, but firm, nurse worked with Danielle for more than an hour to get her to stand up. Getting up off of the bed was hard and painful for Danielle. When we finally got her standing upright, she practically ran down the hall so she could get back into bed as quickly as possible. But when she returned to the room, she was made to sit in the chair for an hour. She was not happy. We followed the same routine the next day. On the fifth day, Dr. Mermelstein advised us that Danielle needed to walk up stairs, so that she could go home "before you catch something from here."

Danielle: When I eventually got back into my hospital bed, I was happy that they took all the IVs out and the other things pertaining to the surgery. Saturday morning, Dr. Mermelstein came in and said, "You are going home, but first you have to be able to walk up and down a flight of stairs." I wondered, "Oh my God, is he crazy?" But I did it.

Once I got home, I walked straight to my bed and took a nap. It took some adjusting to be able to sleep through the night. The biggest problem I had to overcome was getting up from lying down. With some practice, we figured out the easiest way. Everything took a little thought. My friend Samantha came over to sleep for a few days. Having a good friend to keep me company helped a lot.

Mom: It was a long week but I didn't leave her side. After seeing how hard it was to get her up and out of bed in the hospital, I was in sheer panic. So before coming home, her step-dad put her bed in the living room and raised it up, so she didn't have to lower herself down into the bed. We bought a toilet seat riser from the drug store, so that getting up and down from the toilet would not be such a distance. You do not realize the muscles you use in order to do this.

With a spinal fusion for a top curve, it is difficult for someone to twist in order to clean themselves. The shower was a project. We got a shower bench for the tub. I tied a large clean white towel around her neck. I got a hairdresser's plastic cape and put it tightly around her neck so that the water would not seep in and down her back onto her incision. I washed her hair, and she felt good and refreshed.

GIVING BACK

Danielle: A few weeks after my surgery, I was able to attend the next Curvy Girls meeting. I was really looking forward to seeing the girls. They were so happy to see me. I am now proud to say I'm a Curvy Girl. I look forward to helping other girls who need support or just someone to listen to. When scoliosis came into my life, I was afraid. With the help and support from my family and the Curvy Girls, I turned my fears into strength, and was given a new outlook of what giving back was all about.

JENNA

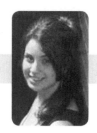

Age: 15

Braced at age 13

I love to design and I'm pursuing a career in fashion. I sew and love to create new things, while incorporating vintage elements into my clothing and accessory designs.

Curvy Girls helped me find the light at the end of the tunnel.

Jenna's Message: Try not to just look at what scoliosis has taken away from you, remember to notice all the gifts it has given you.

When Life Throws You a Curve, Stand Tall

Jenna

I never thought it would happen to me. I foolishly believed things like this only happen to other people. If I were to be honest, I would have to admit I was a bit spoiled. You see, I'm the type of person who always knew what I wanted and set out to get it. I had my whole life planned out in my mind and I was only thirteen. It certainly didn't hurt being an only child and having two great parents who did their best to make my life as comfortable as possible. But having this great life didn't protect me from developing this genetic disease. I guess, in a way, that's what made this diagnosis so difficult to handle.

It had skipped my mother's generation. I was naive to believe I would have been lucky enough to be spared as well. Never did I imagine my life would have changed so completely in the minute it took the doctor to tell me I had scoliosis.

I cried because I was scared and embarrassed at the thought of wearing this plastic back brace to high school. I cried because I knew everything was going to change, and it made me sad. It depressed me to think that I would be different from all the other kids. I wouldn't be able to be a cheerleader, let alone dance anymore.

As I began to adjust to the changes, and start to believe everything was going to be okay, my back brace made me sore and uncomfortable. I felt like I was in the eye of a hurricane, calm before the storm, and then *bam*; I was in pain every day. The brace irritated my skin to the extent that it gave me sores and made me bleed. Wearing the brace twenty-three hours a day was painful physically, spiritually, and emotionally. It was then that I realized the life I knew was gone. My life was now consumed with doctor appointments, yoga lessons, and back brace adjustments, which replaced my dance classes, as well as the after-school activities I used to enjoy.

81

I had to face the inevitable fact that the brace was not going away, and this bulky piece of plastic would accompany me everywhere, including to my favorite retail stores. This led me to the next major problem, wearing a brace to high school. Nothing stylish fit over it. Nothing! This for me was insane because out of all my friends, I was the one who aspired to be a fashion designer one day. I was the one who loved to wear Juicy Couture, shop at Bloomingdale's, and now was forced to resign myself to living in sweats. Wearing this brace made me feel isolated and unattractive. I did my best to alter my baggy clothes but nothing helped. I threw myself into hours of sketching out all my dream clothes. Ironically, as much as I hated my back brace, I didn't dare take it off. I was too scared at the thought of facing surgery, so I wore my brace all the time. I prayed I would never have to face spine surgery.

I became bitter and angry that this had happened to me. After months of being upset, keeping a secret, changing in the bathroom for gym, and wearing extra baggy clothes, I decided there was no need to keep this up. I came to peace with having scoliosis, and I was ready to face anyone who had something to say about it. I was confident now that I wouldn't burst into tears if someone asked me if I needed surgery; I would be able to answer calmly. Unfortunately, the sad truth was, at that point, I really didn't know what the outcome was going to be. I just prayed that surgery would never be an option for me.

Regrettably, that feeling of peace only lasted so long. The stress of having a chronic condition wore me down mentally, and to make matters worse, I didn't have many friends to support me through my treatment. I quickly learned who my real friends were and weren't. It was a shock that the one person I trusted the most, let me down the most in the end. I soon learned that I could not rely on others, only myself.

I think what upset me the most was that no one understood what I was going through or even had an ounce of compassion. Many thought I was embellishing or I just wanted attention. My favorite was that I was used to being spoiled, and I just wanted special treatment. Didn't they know that I didn't want this? Didn't they know that what I wanted desperately was to blend in, and not be different? I felt like everyone was watching me all the time and it made me panic-stricken. Panic disorder was the aftermath of my scoliosis. To this day, I still feel panicky in certain environments. Near the end of my treatment, I couldn't take it. I lost it. I began to lose faith, and began questioning if everything I had given up these last several years would be worth it in the end.

Happily, the brace treatment worked! I got my wish. I will never be straight, but that's okay. I am just as beautiful as I was before I had scoliosis. Maybe even more, because I am "curvy" now.

> I have come to peace with my uneven hips, and how my spine curves like a backward "S."

I am not the same eighth-grade girl that was concerned with looking into her Chanel compact. I have more depth. There was a time I only saw what scoliosis had taken away from me, but now that my treatment is over, I can look back on what having scoliosis has given me. I discovered that our obstacles are our greatest teachers. Scoliosis made my love for fashion much deeper, brought out my creativity, and forced me to become more innovative. Trying to create outfits to hide my brace led me to begin taking fashion classes in school, and art classes in the evening. I learned not to falter, to rely on myself, and to find inspiration within. This road was part of the journey that made me who I am today. My favorite author Emily Giffin writes, "Sometimes the absolute last thing you want is the one thing you need."

The lessons I learned from battling scoliosis, no one could have taught me. I had to figure them out on my own.

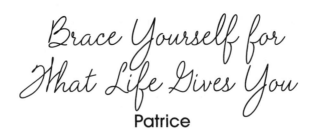

Brace Yourself for What Life Gives You

Patrice

In 1949, my mother had spinal fusion surgery. The surgery is nothing like what they do today. In those days, surgeons didn't have titanium rods; instead, bone was taken from the child's leg to fuse the spine together. As if the surgery itself wasn't difficult enough, she was put in a body cast that encompassed her entire torso, from her chest to her lower hips. Once she was able to leave the hospital, she was sent to a convalescent home for nearly a year, due to the amount of rehabilitation she needed. You can only imagine how difficult this was for a child to go through at only twelve years old.

As a young girl, I'll never forget the first time I saw my mother's back. It was horrible. It was terribly crooked and the scarring looked like railroad tracks. While her physical scars were quite visible, her emotional scarring, though hidden, impacted her just as much.

Growing up, I was always reminded about my mother's scoliosis because it prevented her from doing a lot of things with my brother and I. Sadly, I was never told that this could have been a hereditary disease. And I had no reason to think otherwise since neither my brother nor I had any trace of scoliosis. I think this is where my guilt began. I should have known. Why did I have to find out the hard way that scoliosis can skip a generation? How did I get spared and yet my daughter wasn't? Why didn't I know?

It started the day Jenna was trying on a new bathing suit. She dropped a tag and as she bent over to pick it up, I saw it. I saw the "hump." Oh my God! I knew immediately. It was scoliosis. I didn't say anything. Trying to remain calm I asked Jenna to bend over again, and sure enough there it was. All I kept thinking was that Jenna was the same age my mother was when she had spinal surgery; this can't be happening. And yet, in an instant, all the pieces began to fit together.

I began to recall the prior year when Jenna had complained of hip pain. She stopped participating in some of her gym activities at school which we had just chalked up to her being a preteen and a (little) bit lazy. When she told us that she was getting "sharp, shooting pains," we realized that laziness had nothing to do with it and immediately took her to the pediatrician. She found nothing seriously wrong and shrugged it off to growing pains. In hindsight, an x-ray should have been taken since scoliosis was written in Jenna's family medical history.

I remembered thinking there was something wrong with Jenna's left foot, as it turned slightly inward. Again, I brought this to the pediatrician's attention, but my concerns were dismissed. I would later learn that this was related to her scoliosis.

Jenna, ironically, passed all the scoliosis screenings at school and even passed the yearly school physical. This also upset me because, in retrospect, her pediatrician should have been monitoring her more closely, especially at this age when scoliosis usually makes its appearance.

Not having an answer as to why she had ribcage pain and the shooting pains in her hip, she developed a lot of anxiety. She imagined that something more serious was wrong, something like cancer. It would take the diagnosis from the specialist to help calm things down.

I didn't bother taking her back to the pediatrician; I knew she needed to go straight to a specialist. Like all of us, when you know your child has a serious health issue, you research for the best. Our best brought us into Manhattan. After Jenna's evaluation, the doctor immediately said she had a double major curve and a kyphosis—an outward curve causing a hunching of the upper spine; something that she probably inherited from her grandmother and her great-grandmother. Hearing that it was scoliosis helped Jenna in one respect, but it also ignited a new set of anxieties. She feared she would end up needing spinal surgery like her grandmother.

Since Jenna's curves were already in the 30s, her treatment plan was standard—bracing for twenty-three hours a day, seven days a week for an untold amount of time. Listening to their plan of treatment felt as if I was punched in the stomach. I couldn't believe what I was hearing. Poor Jenna just gasped and my husband Kenny just stood in silence. How quickly the atmosphere in the doctor's office changed. A minute ago, my fashionista daughter was giggling while waiting for the doctor to come in, all the while designing a couture dress from the blue paper gown she was wearing. It took just one minute from the time he entered the exam room to change our upbeat moods to sadness and tears.

Once he left, we were all speechless, shocked, and numb. I heard this nonstop voice whispering, "This can't be happening." How did the scoliosis skip my generation and affect Jenna? Nothing made sense. I thought we were in the clear once scoliosis passed me by.

The longer we thought about the reality of the situation, the bleaker things seemed to get. As if the diagnosis wasn't bad enough, Jenna was entering her first year of high school in the fall. How was she supposed to wear this brace to school? All I did was cry. It killed me that she had to be going through all this.

Two weeks later, the brace was ready to be picked up. Jenna was a trooper; she had good and bad days. When her days were bad, I'd find her crying, so I would just tell her to take it off. I couldn't bear seeing her in so much physical and emotional pain from this brace. But as much as Jenna hated to wear the brace, the fear of an operation was even more terrifying. I know I was wrong to tell her to take the brace off, but I was frustrated for her. I wanted to take her pain and sadness away even if it was just for a little while. Thankfully, Jenna didn't listen to me. Her fear of surgery was the driving force to compliancy.

We were lucky in one way that we had the summer to gradually adjust to bracing without the pressure of being in school. As the school year approached, we spent our days shopping for clothes that were stylish, comfortable and *hid* the brace. We learned early on how challenging shopping for clothes was going to be. Jenna's brace was big and since it had the straps going over her shoulder for her kyphosis, it made it more difficult to find tops to cover this ugly barbaric brace. Who would have ever thought that my daughter who loved to shop for clothes would find shopping physically and emotionally exhausting?

As the days progressed, we decided to take things one step at a time. First, she would need to deal with the challenges of wearing a hard plastic brace that was hot and stiff on her body 23/7. She was given a tee shirt to wear under her brace in order to prevent any skin irritation. Unfortunately for Jenna, the tee shirts didn't help to prevent the chaffing and sores that were to follow.

Once school began, Jenna did a great job of wearing her brace to school every day. Our school district was very generous in all the support they gave Jenna through these very difficult years. A special education teacher, Deena Stevens, helped me to implement a 504 plan that accommodated Jenna's need to wear a back brace during school. Jenna was provided with two lockers, one of which was big enough for her to put her brace in when she needed to take it off. In the beginning, she did this often because she would break out in a sweat from becoming overheated in her "plastic sauna." The school provided fans and air-conditioning wherever it was available. She was given an elevator pass and extra time to get to her classes, since walking up and down the stairs was awkward.

We thought we had everything in place for a successful school year, until Jenna met with a major friend disappointment. On top of all the garbage our girls go through physically and psychologically, they have to learn like everyone else who their true friends are and how unfair life can be. Once again my heart broke for Jenna; she didn't deserve this. Normally, kids at this age feel like they can get through almost anything as long as they have their friends to talk things over with. But what happens when a friend decides to abandon you?

> No one prepares you as a parent
> to help your child through
> this emotional roller coaster,
> let alone with a diagnosis of scoliosis.

I decided to guide Jenna toward her creative passion for fashion drawing and design. I wanted to keep her distracted from the pain of losing her friend and not being physically able to keep up with her other friends. I enrolled her in a fine arts program and kept her busy with sewing and drawing lessons.

However, through all the let downs, Jenna also learned she had a devoted father, who went to every doctor's appointment and stood by her side every night encouraging her as she did her very painful kyphosis exercises. She also learned she had a wonderful support team at school. Her teachers and the school nurses were there for her when I couldn't be.

We continued with our routine orthopedic visits. Jenna went to all her appointments prepared with questions. It saddened me because I strongly disliked Jenna's orthopedic physician. She was indifferent and cold-mannered. She had a way of making me feel combative because of her lack of empathy. I guess she thought she needed to be like this in order to have her patients comply with her recommended therapy.

When Jenna was diagnosed with scoliosis, she would spend hours reading and researching this disease on the Internet. During one of her searches, she came across an announcement about a walk being held at Jones Beach by the Scoliosis Association of Long Island. I contacted the person in charge and she invited us to attend. We decided to go with the hope we might meet other families going through the same issues we were. Unfortunately, when we got there we didn't see many people at all. I looked around and said, "This is it?"

Jenna took her friends for a walk hoping to meet others with scoliosis, while I waited. I stood there just staring at the ocean and truly feeling depressed. I had hoped we would have met other young families who had scoliosis, but there weren't any. I remembered just staring out into this endless ocean of blue water and saying, "Please God, I need your help. You need to help us get through this." A few minutes later Jenna came running towards me with a flyer in her hands. It said, "My name is Leah. I'm 14 and I'm starting a Kid's Scoliosis Group." I looked around but there was nobody to be seen. It was as if the flyer came from the sky.

"Look," said Jenna, "there's a girl who started a support group for scoliosis. She's like me."

I wanted to cry. I just looked up and said, "Thank you."

Meeting Robin and Leah along with all the other families was wonderful. This was exactly what we needed. Leah held the meetings for the girls downstairs, while Robin held meetings for parents upstairs. The parent meeting allowed all of us to discuss openly our personal fears without worrying that our daughters could hear us. These meetings helped get us through a very difficult time.

Presently, Jenna is being weaned from her brace after two years. Her scoliosis is the best it could be. She did everything right. She compliantly wore her brace and her curve not only stopped progressing, but we managed to get a curve reduction into the twenties. Today, Jenna still has to do her kyphosis exercises and since she is being weaned, she only has to wear her brace at night to sleep. The worst is over and now it's about appreciating all the people in your life who helped you get through this difficult time.

Robin Stoltz will always have a special place in my heart. She was there for my daughter and me, helping us through so many challenges. There are some people in our lives that will come and go, but I truly believe that the friendships we made with the original Curvy Girls support group members will last us a lifetime.

DEANNA

Age: 14

Braced at age 13

I wear a lot of bracelets. I like to sing, act, read, and write, spend time with my friends and family, attend youth group, listen to music, and play piano.

Curvy Girls has helped me to get through my scoliosis experience, and lets me pass on what I've gotten out of it to girls who are going through the same thing.

Deanna's Message: Have a friend come over to help you decide which clothes look best for your brace.

"Claire"

Deanna

I was eleven when they detected a small curve in my spine. It was never really a big deal, because the curve was only about 9°. To make sure it didn't get worse, every four months I'd go back to an orthopedic doctor to have my back x-rayed.

About a week after my thirteenth birthday, we went back for a scheduled follow-up appointment. The wait to get in to see the doctor was always endless. During that time, my mom pointed out a girl who was wearing a back brace for scoliosis. As I casually glanced over, I couldn't help but think how hard it must be for her.

Finally, our names were called. Once in the exam room, I quickly changed into my paper gown and was taken down the hall for x-rays. A few minutes later, I returned to the room and waited for the doctor. When she entered, she smiled and offered me a lollipop, and then proceeded to give us bad news. She told us that my curves had increased, and she believed it would be beneficial at this point for me to be braced before my curves became worse. I immediately flashed back to the girl from the waiting room. I looked over to my mom in disbelief, and the two of us just broke down and cried.

I was so upset and frustrated. I was upset with the unexpected news of finding out that I needed to wear a back brace. Then I wondered why in the world the doctor would think that giving a lollipop to a thirteen-year-old would cheer her up after finding out this awful news. I couldn't believe this was happening. I already felt like there were so many things wrong with me. I had to wear contact lenses, my orthodontic braces were put on, and now they're telling me I have to wear a back brace for sixteen hours a day. Was I starting to feel sorry for myself? I wasn't quite sure until I came home from the doctor's office only to find out I got my period for the first time! Could things get any worse?

A week later, I had my first appointment with the "brace-makers." Measurements were taken so that my brace would be molded to fit me specifically. The orthotist who was taking the measurements insisted that I suck in my breath. I was very uncomfortable, but did exactly what I was told.

Once the brace was finished, my whole family went to the office to pick it up. They watched me put the brace on, and I couldn't help but notice that it looked and felt like I was in a hard-shelled corset. Having my parents yank the straps caused me so much pain; all I could do was cry.

Because I was in so much pain, my parents started looking into an alternative brace called the SpineCor®. This brace was different. It wasn't made of hard plastic like the Boston Brace. Instead it was made of cloth and straps that wrap around your body. But before we could go any further, my parents decided to get a second opinion.

Unfortunately, when we went for the second opinion we didn't exactly hear what we had hoped. The new orthopedist explained that the SpineCor® brace would not be as effective for me as the Boston Brace. In addition, to get the best results from bracing, he said I needed to be braced for twenty-three hours a day, not the sixteen hours originally prescribed. My hopes of getting out of wearing my hard brace were crushed.

After this appointment, my parents and I agreed that we wanted to change doctors. Dr. Hargovind Dewal sent us to his orthotist to see if he could make some adjustments to my current brace. This guy was great. He loosened the brace, making it so I could actually breathe, and assured me that it would still be effective. It was then that I realized this might not be so bad.

There was good news and bad news. The bad news was that I had to wear the back brace during school. The good news was that my mom took me on a shopping spree for new clothes to cover the brace! When we were done shopping, I invited my best friend over for support. I showed her everything I bought and tried it on. Having a friend tell you when the brace could be seen under my new clothes turned into something fun.

Gradually, I became more and more comfortable wearing my brace, probably because I had such great support from my friends. I remember this one time when I was hanging out with my three best friends, Amanda, Blaine, and David. We were in Amanda's backyard, when Blaine took my brace and sat under the trampoline. It was there she decided to give my brace a name. We all just laughed. When Blaine finally came out from under the trampoline, my brace was officially named Claire.

As time went on, Blaine and Amanda continued to support me with Claire. I definitely believe it was their support that helped me wear my brace for twenty-three hours every day. I no longer had to worry about hiding Claire. Whether we were in gym class, rehearsals for plays, or just hanging out with friends, I was confident and comfortable enough to take Claire off and leave her out in the open, as well as wear her over my clothes. Sometimes it served as a conversation starter, a tickle guard, or even a mascot.

> To be honest, I felt the brace
> had become a part of me,
> a part of my personality.

After wearing my brace for a year, I actually looked forward to my next doctor's appointment. My family and I were feeling hopeful that there might be a chance the doctor would begin to wean me off the brace. Sadly, this was not the case. He didn't want to take any chances of my curves getting worse when we were so close to the end.

My parents were so upset. I felt disappointed, but the weird thing was that I couldn't picture myself without my brace, no matter how much of a pain it was. So it wasn't the end of the world when Dr. Dewal said, "A couple more months."

We left the office and went to a diner to get something to eat. When the waiter came to take our order, we were all crying. I felt kind of stupid but I wanted to tell my parents that I wasn't mentally ready to get rid of my brace. When I finally spoke up, I think they understood. I felt like if it weren't for my brace, I wouldn't have found my own personality. Instead, I probably would have just followed whatever my friends did. I still had some self-discovery to do.

During the next six months, so many things changed in my life. I was having problems with friends, both new and old. I was going on a retreat with my youth group, starting high school, and I had a new haircut. My closest friends and family continued to support me, but I felt something change. It was my brace. I was getting fed up with wearing it.

I was starting to get tired of all the questions and annoying little quirks that came with my brace. The limited clothing I was able to wear frustrated me. The gym lockers were much smaller in the high school, which meant I had to leave my brace in the gym teacher's office. I can't wear my brace when I sing, which I had to do for two straight periods of music.

After a year and a half of being strong about the whole "brace situation," I broke down and started crying. I was ready to give it up! I didn't know how I'd continue to brace if things went bad at my next appointment. I was frustrated and needed to finally vent all my fears that I had kept inside.

The day of the appointment I had my entire family there for support. After waiting for what seemed like ages, the doctor came in and said, that although I was not ready to completely wean off the brace, he could allow me to not wear it during school. This was the news I was waiting to hear. I was so happy! When we left, we went back to that same diner as we did after my last appointment. This time we were celebrating!

All my friends were so happy for me. I think the only "bad" thing about not wearing my brace during school is that I am extremely ticklish and now I don't have my "tickle guard!"

As for now, I hope that within the next couple of months I'll begin to wean even more from wearing my brace. This has been a crazy, life-changing experience, but without it I don't think I'd be myself.

My Daughter Makes Me Cry

Marianne

It started out as a routine office visit, when our pediatrician first discovered that my eleven-year-old daughter, Deanna, had a slight curve in her spine. Keeping on the safe side, my doctor thought it would be a good idea for us to see an orthopedic spine specialist. I wasn't too concerned. We scheduled the appointment with a highly recommended orthopedic specialist. At Deanna's first visit, I went prepared with a list of questions: "How would scoliosis affect my daughter's day-to-day routine?" "Would she outgrow it?" "Did we need to possibly have her start some kind of physical therapy?"

To our surprise, after the x-rays were completed, the doctor informed us that Deanna had two curves, which meant that her tiny back was growing in an "S" shape. With her fistful of lollipops, the doctor explained that Deanna had a 9° curve on the top and a 7° curve on the bottom. However, since scoliosis is not diagnosed until after 10°, there was no treatment recommended at this time. We were to return for monitoring every four months. She added that, with a little luck, once Deanna began her menstrual cycle, she would soon stop growing and there would be no need to consider further treatment.

As Deanna was growing into a beautiful teenager, I couldn't help but hope that maybe she'd be tall like her Aunt Gina, and thin like her mom. Over the course of the next year, when Deanna grew nearly six inches, I began to notice changes in her spine.

The next two office visits were quite the same. I asked about physical therapy. The doctor candidly told us that we could try, but it wasn't proven to help scoliosis. Over the next four months, we tried physical therapy. At our appointment, the therapist noticed a significant discrepancy in the length of Deanna's legs and recommended putting in a shoe lift. I refused until I could speak to her orthopedist. I was unaware, at that time, that discrepancy in leg length may be a sign of scoliosis.

I hoped it was a good sign when Deanna's appointment fell on her birthday, April 4th. Maybe we would leave in celebration. We chose an earlier appointment time, figuring that the wait wouldn't be as horrendous as it usually was. To help distract us, I began to talk to Deanna about the play in which she had just landed a role. A part of me was listening to her talk, and the other part was getting lost in my own thoughts. I kept wishing, "I hope this is the last time we'll be sitting in this room."

Deanna was taken for x-rays. She returned with a smile and was greeted by the doctor with her fistful of lollipops. This time, though, the doctor wore a different expression. She asked Deanna to stand so she could measure her arm span and height. Deanna had grown two more inches since our last visit. I thought this was good, but no one spoke. It was too quiet. The doctor popped the x-ray up on the computer and, much to my surprise, there it was, my daughter's crooked little spine. I tried everything in my power not to cry. I knew then that this was not going to be our last visit.

After a long pause, the doctor gave us the bad news. In the past four months, Deanna's curve jumped from 15° on the top, to 27°, and her lower curve progressed from 20° to 31°. There would be no other choice but to brace her, and hope that we would be able to contain or stop the curve from progressing any further. Deanna immediately began to cry. I tried my best to keep my composure while asking the right questions. I needed to be able to take all this in so I could help my daughter understand that this was the only option. Dr. H. instructed me on what I needed to do. I called my husband, Kevin, as soon as we left.

Being a close family, Kevin felt terrible that he wasn't with us when we found out such shocking news. He immediately focused on what we needed to do, and that was to schedule an appointment with an orthotist for a brace. Once that was taken care of, we would return for another x-ray taken in the brace to make sure it fit correctly.

Deanna, my husband, my son, and I went together to the orthotist appointment. A man came into the small room and began to fit Deanna for her brace. One of the first things he asked her to do was take a deep breath so that the brace would fit her snug. Watching the orthotist work on Deanna made me feel helpless. All I could do was sit and cry.

Waiting for the brace to be completed gave me more time to think. I had so many questions running through my head. One of my biggest concerns was Deanna's self-esteem. As a teenager, how would it be for her to wear this brace to school? What if she was made fun of or excluded from activities because of this brace? Kids can be so mean and girls can be the cruelest! These were all thoughts I knew Deanna must be agonizing over, but was keeping them to herself. I was concerned about how she would sleep at night in that brace. Then I realized that there was something I could do to help. We'd get her the most comfortable mattress we could find. I just wish we could have solved all her problems as quickly and easily.

Before we knew it, we were back at the orthotist's office to experience yet another horrendous visit. When they put Deanna into the new brace, she had difficulty taking in a deep breath. She couldn't sit because the brace was so tight. How would she be able to sleep in this? Looking at her struggling, both my husband and I wondered if there might be an alternative. It seemed such a barbaric way to treat scoliosis in this day and age.

Kevin researched and found another form of bracing called the SpineCor®. He spent that day and night speaking with professionals about this brace made of cloth and straps. We were hoping to try and purchase it so that Deanna wouldn't be tortured by wearing her current brace. When we went to confer with Dr. H. about writing a prescription for the SpineCor®, we were seen instead by her physician assistant (PA). Deanna put on the Boston Brace to be x-rayed and she began to cry. Both my husband and I pleaded with all our heart to convince the PA that this brace was not perfect for Deanna, and that a brace like the SpineCor® would be a better solution. The PA did not concur; however, she did agree to give us a prescription as long as we understood that this was not what she recommended.

When she left the room to get us the new prescription, Deanna broke down crying, saying, "How am I supposed to do this? Why ME? It's not fair!!" When the PA returned and heard how upset Deanna was, she scolded her, "Deanna, you need to just deal with this. It's not your parent's fault, so stop this now!" My arms were folded across my chest and my fists were ready to punch this woman. How dare she speak to my daughter with such disregard? In her profession, how could she not understand how difficult this is for a twelve-year-old child? Regrettably, I said nothing. I just took our new prescription, left, and never returned.

The Boston Brace lay in the backseat of my car until we were able to further investigate the SpineCor® brace. In the meantime, Deanna was trying to accept that she would need to wear some kind of brace. We decided to obtain a second opinion before pursuing this further.

We went to Long Island Spine Specialists, hoping that the doctor would approve of the SpineCor®. After reviewing all of Deanna's x-rays, he agreed that Deanna needed to be braced. He explained that because her curve was already above 24°, she was not a candidate for SpineCor®. It was decided. We were resigned to staying with the Boston Brace.

What we liked about this orthopedist was that he seemed to have everything we were looking for in a doctor. He had his facts and was precise. Most importantly, he was sympathetic. Dr. Dewal continued to explain that Deanna needed to wear the Boston Brace, but he believed she needed to be braced for twenty-three hours a day and not sixteen hours. As far as the brace we currently owned, Dr. Dewal suggested it be refitted by his orthotist. That evening, when we left his office, something had changed. Maybe we were all beginning to accept bracing as our *only* option.

We met with our new orthotist, Mike, who readjusted Deanna's brace with both care and concern for her comfort. He felt confident that he would make this brace work for her. Mike explained to us that he too had been diagnosed with scoliosis as a child. He proceeded to give Deanna tips on wearing the brace, specifically, how to sit and bend. From that day on, Deanna was compliant and wore her brace twenty-three hours a day for the next year and ten months.

At our follow-up visit with Dr. Dewal, we hoped this would be the day Deanna could begin weaning from her brace. She was x-rayed and measured. We learned that she grew an inch from the prior visit. We also found out that the straps on her brace needed to be replaced, a sure sign of brace wear compliance! The good news was that her curve did not progress, but because her growth plate had not yet closed (Risser 3 out of 5), she would need to continue to wear her brace. When I realized that she would have to start high school wearing a brace, I couldn't speak for fear I would cry. Maybe luck would come at our next office visit. After all, it was scheduled on my birthday.

We drove in silence to a nearby diner for lunch. As we sat there, Deanna amazed me once again. She wanted to know if I was all right. She told me I shouldn't cry and explained, "Mommy, this brace defines me, and I'm not ready to give it up yet!" When I think about that moment, I realize how lucky I am to be blessed with such an amazing daughter.

We didn't get to go on my birthday after all, because the day of our appointment was changed. Was this a good omen or bad? There we were, Kevin, Deanna, Anthony, and I, same procedure. Deanna left to be x-rayed, and then returned to wait with us. Dr. Dewal walked in to see us all waiting with our fingers, arms, legs, and toes crossed, hoping to hear "good" news. He told us that Deanna had once again not progressed and that her Risser was now a 4, meaning her growth plate has almost closed. But he didn't mention weaning, so my husband asked, "What about increasing her time out of the brace for the seven hours of school?" I held my breath, as I'm sure Deanna did. He contemplated and then agreed. We left that day jumping and screaming with tears of joy! We returned to that same diner, but this time for a celebratory dinner!

Four months later, Deanna's scoliosis had still not progressed. We credit this to her strict discipline of bracing. She has been supported by a wonderful group of friends and family. There are times I look at her in awe because she is so secure with herself. Without complaint, she was able to wear this brace to bed, school, vacations, and even wore it over her clothes. She never felt she had to hide it from the world. Deanna makes me so proud just knowing she was able to handle this enormous challenge. My daughter makes me cry!

OLIVIA "LIV"

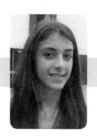

Age: 13

Braced at age 12

I like to listen to music and I read a lot of books. I also like fashion design.

Curvy Girls is a good support group. I can vent my angry feelings about the brace and have people that understand because they have been through what I am currently going through. It's nice to have people there when your parents don't understand.

Liv's Message: Don't pretend you can handle all the changes you are going through by yourself.

My Life Sucks!

"Liv"

Scoliosis has changed me. It changed the way I view myself and how I act. I used to be a shy girl with fluffy brown hair, dark eye circles, a crooked neck, and a yellow shirt with beads falling off the collar. I wore that shirt every day since being fitted into what I still consider a trap. This feeling has not left me since my doctor first molded me. Being crammed into something so tight and visible was difficult. To be honest, it hasn't gotten much better.

While I've become less ashamed around my friends, I still get nervous about being bumped or touched by strangers or cute boys, fearing that they would judge me. I am a little shallow like that. I began to wear makeup and straighten my hair. I cried and cried until my mom let me buy my own hair straightening iron. Crying was what I did best ever since I got my brace. I stopped drawing manga, a Japanese form of cartoon characters. I soon stopped wearing the ugly yellow shirt and got into my cell phone, boys, hair, clothes, and shoes. Who was I? Who had I become?

It felt like overnight I had begun to mature, or so I thought. At some point, I started to handle my brace a little differently. Sometimes I left it on all day, afraid if I didn't, that karma might just slap me in the face. Then there were the other days that I didn't care about the "karma," and I would go to the gym locker room and shove my brace in the locker until my day ended.

Once I became "pretty," I seemed to gain even more friends. Guys talked to me and my close friends began to respect me a little more. Life with the brace began to seem more manageable. The thing that really saved me was the summer before I became "normal." While at summer camp I became "popular." I had a lot of friends and they all loved me, and yet I still hadn't told anyone about my brace.

During camp, we went to my friend's Bat Mitzvah. I went to the bathroom to loosen my brace, when my friends asked me where I was going. The words just spilled out of my mouth, "To loosen my brace."

I proceeded to explain everything to them. Much to my surprise, they were sympathetic and kind. They supported me through all of it. Soon everyone at camp knew about my brace and I was even respected for it. My friends didn't care about what was plastered to my body. I assumed then that these were friends that would stay in my life for a while.

That fall, when I returned to school all pretty, kids instantly liked me. This was a little embarrassing because I wanted to be liked for me, not for what I looked like. I became a little more outgoing, and I realized my friends did appreciate my personality. It made me feel good.

Then one day, I broke down. It was my first breakdown of the new school year. I didn't want to feel different, and yet I did. How could I not when everyone had nice bodies and was able to wear pretty clothes, while I was stuck with three lumpy straps poking out of my back and giant hips?

"!#*?!" I cried to myself, repeating the word over and over. I felt like my life was at a breaking point and it would all disappear. So I waited. Nothing changed. My back had giant curves from the mistakes that my first and second doctors made.

⁓

I'm now seeing a third doctor. He's working out okay, I guess. But I still have the brace. Having this contraption stuck on me is getting really annoying, and every second of my life, I want to rip this thing off and burn it. But I can't and I won't. It sucks though, being trapped.

Nobody, not my parents nor my friends, truly understand how much this affects and defines me. I can't help but wonder how my life would've gone if this brace never existed. I constantly have to squat to pick up things off the floor. I wish people could see what I really look like. I want so many things.

Honestly, I hate my parents all the time. I hate my friends all the time. They act like they care, like they understand, but they don't. I'm sure at times they try, but they never will understand how much this affects me. I wish words could describe the pain I get from putting on the brace every morning, and the relief I get from taking it off even for two seconds, when nobody's watching.

I do soccer and track and I work out every Saturday. I am trying to be like other people with the brace. I don't know if it's working, but I'm getting there. Inch by inch, one rung up the ladder at a time, and I'm halfway to the top. The problem is that I don't want to be halfway. I want to be at the top. Unfortunately, my journey is not complete. Sometimes you just have to throw your hands up in the air and yell, "SCREW IT!" But to be truthful, that doesn't help at all; it just relieves a little stress. Then, I cry. I always cry. Crying hurts so bad and feels so good. It's twisted and unnerving, but sometimes, maybe even all the time, I need to. The best I can do is walk with my head held high and smile like I don't give a damn, even though I give the biggest damn of all.

Welcome to the Scoli-Jungle

Judith

Our little 15-pound doggie, Bessie, has scoliosis. If you trace her spine with your finger, you will feel an "S" instead of a straight line. So, she runs in a crooked line and sometimes cannot jump onto her usual chairs and beds. Otherwise, if we put round silver framed glasses on her, she'd be a ringer for Jerry Garcia. She continues to toss her kibbles in attempts to engage us in "soccer kibble" games, taunt our 90-pound dog, and pick the choicest spots to sleep, roll in, and eat yucky stuff.

Our ten-year-old daughter, on the other hand, has a cervical curve, plus a backward "S" curve. I recently discovered that the degrees of Liv's curves vary greatly according to each doctor, as they all seem to read her x-ray measurements at different vertebrae.

Liv began treatment at a hospital in Manhattan with her mid-thoracic and lumbar curves at 25°. She was Boston-braced (molded to her body, not padded) by a "top" pediatric orthopedic surgeon, who seemed to hand out scripts for CAT scans to his patients like candy. Needless to say, stuffing a ten-year-old claustrophobic kid into one of those machines without earplugs or music is quite horrific. Especially when the first machine ended up breaking mid-scan, and poor Liv had to start all over on another machine. Thankfully, the second technician did not understand English very well, and kept hysterically laughing away Liv's pleas for release. A forty-five-minute procedure ended up taking four hours.

Liv wore her Boston Brace, despite open sores, welts, and bruising. She rarely complained even in the heat of summer. When I called the orthotist and pediatric orthopedic surgeon about the skin irritations, they BOTH said to apply rubbing alcohol to "toughen up her skin." Why would anyone put rubbing alcohol on open sores? Instead, Liv faithfully applied Ammens® powder and gauze pads and still did not complain.

We saw the pediatric orthopedic surgeon during the summer, and he did not change his opinion about the brace, abruptly dismissing

Liv's reports of back pain. Meanwhile, I took Liv to see two other pediatric orthopedic surgeons for consultations—only to learn at the surgeon's office that one of them did not even see kids with scoliosis. That was most disheartening, especially after office staff had previously assured me that the surgeon did see kids. This lack of communication cost us greatly, since my insurance only covered one pediatric consult per year.

Finally, the pain was so bad that Liv started crying, so I took pictures of her skin and showed the pediatric orthopedic surgeon at her follow-up visit. Liv stayed in the same brace for nine months while she grew over two inches. First, the pediatric orthopedic surgeon said that Liv should not be growing so fast. (Huh?) Second, he said that there was no significant change in her curves. Despite my request, he did not go over the x-rays with me. Third, he said that Liv was due for a new brace and should stop wearing the present one immediately. It would take at least two weeks to make a new one, and more time off from work and school to schlep back into Manhattan from Long Island to see the orthotist (at his convenience, of course!).

Well, Liv freaked. FREAKED. Absolutely, totally FREAKED OUT right there in the exam room. Naturally, our two minutes were used up, so the doctor was gone before we could ask any more questions. Liv trained herself to tolerate wearing this brace for twenty hours a day for nine months, and was suddenly being told to take it off completely for the next two- to three-weeks. After nine months, this brace became her second skin, her security blanket, literally her backbone. Liv felt like she no longer had a safety net. And here I am, shaking in anger and not being able to speak. Powerless and unable to help take away her emotional hurt or make her feel better physically, I watched this poor kid lose it.

So, my brave daughter decided herself to keep the damn thing on.

SPINECOR®

That night, my husband, Jeff, and I decided to "bite the bullet" and totally abandon the traditional/conservative medical model and stray away from pediatric orthopedic surgeons. Liv was excited to try the flexible brace, which promised more movement, more shopping, and of course, the ability to wear cool jeans. The next day, I called a chiropractor in Manhattan on the recommendation of Liv's current chiropractor to discuss the SpineCor® brace.

After ten months with the molded Boston Brace and 10° later, we switched Liv to the SpineCor®. At this point, Liv had significant scarring from the molded brace.

In fifth grade, the kids ignored the brace. But sixth grade presented her with more of a social and physical challenge. Since Liv didn't want anyone to know about her brace, she went to the nurse's office to change for gym. In seventh grade, she dressed in the locker room stalls, but waited for everyone to leave in order to hide the brace in a locker.

I had worked with my local school district to craft a 504 Plan for Liv. A "504 Plan" helps a child with special health care needs to fully participate in school. This plan enabled me to put in place certain provisions, specifically tailored for her needs during these bracing years. One of the important issues was to allow Liv to be excused from being late to class after gym. Unfortunately, Liv refused to take advantage of what had been set up for her because she didn't want to feel different from the other kids.

I have regularly brought Liv to a chiropractor near our house who is an amazing hands-on healer. He devised a program of strengthening and stretching muscles called Posturcise® that Liv has been using. With the patience and encouragement of her trainer, Dee Dee, Liv can now turn her neck from side-to-side, balance much better, walk straighter. She has also gained more muscle awareness and strength. But after months of her Posturcise® exercises, Liv grew tired of the regimen and devised her own alternative with the help of her trainer. She began doing weight training to increase her overall body strength and encourage straight posture.

Liv is having a harder time with her scoliosis than little Bessie but she is determined to succeed. She continues to wear her brace even though it's never easy. The new one makes it harder for her to sleep, run, or go to the bathroom. She has to find shirts to accommodate the new brace, both for underneath and on top. She mostly keeps her anger in, but clearly feels different from the other kids. It doesn't help that she is also 5 feet 3 inches at age eleven—taller than all of her friends, and me, too. ("Sit down when I yell at you, so I can actually see your eyes!")

Today, I am so proud and surprised by Liv for sharing and showing her new brace with the other Curvy Girls. Normally quiet and observant, Liv even discussed the pros and cons of this brace with the group!

AND LIFE GOES ON

How many people have I spoken to who have scoliosis or know someone who has been braced or even casted (way back when), or who had the surgery themselves? I've lost track. And yet how easy for me to get lost in Liv's journey, which seems all-consuming sometimes.

As it turns out, the SpineCor® was inappropriate for Liv, because her curves were in the mid-30s when she started this regime. I felt as if I had been misled by a fuddy-duddy chiropractor who kept selling me gadgets for Liv to use at home. I now understand that the SpineCor® is better for curves in the low 20s, but Dr. Fuddy-Duddy insisted that it would be great for Liv's curves.

Thank goodness for the Curvy Girls. We received many helpful doctor and orthotist recommendations and critiques. At the end, we went with Leah and Robin's dynamic duo, Dr. Mermelstein and orthotist, Mike Mangino. Jeff and I decided not to see them originally because Dr. Mermelstein was not in our insurance plan.

I have now learned that "top-rated" doctors are not necessarily that, especially with regard to bedside manner! I was determined to have both—competence and compassion in a surgeon. This, in addition to the lack of scoli-braced-qualified in-network doctors, led us to Dr. Mermelstein's doorstep in Commack. First, Dr. Mermelstein has evening hours, which means no more taking off work and school for appointments. A real relief for working moms! Second, the instant we walked into the office, everyone was genuinely warm.

The x-rays showed that her curves grew more and were at 39° and 41°, creeping toward surgery. So another Boston Brace was prescribed, to which Liv and I complained loudly. Dr. Mermelstein explained that this one is made only with Liv's body measurements, with pads inserted to challenge her curve. Her first brace required that she lay on a weird contraption and have her body wrapped in Plaster of Paris, which dried on her body, and was then sawed off. We did not know what to expect from this new brace.

We visited Mike Mangino, and in two weeks, we had a brace that was really different than her first one. This brace actually looked comfortable, and holy cow, Liv could do the straps herself. She did not lose color when she put it on, and she could sit and breathe in it. This brace had air holes in the front, gave a little if she leaned forward, and it didn't come up so high on the sides. An added bonus, Mike Mangino's office said my insurance paid entirely for the brace and all office visits for him. Another wow!

But of course, she doesn't want to wear it and she doesn't want anyone to know. The nurse at school has called me at work, concerned that Liv isn't wearing her brace enough. I know she isn't. I know she wears it too loosely in bed. She knows the risks, especially since Jeff and I remind her frequently. I started saving for surgery, though sometimes I feel guilty, hoping that I am not "jinxing" Liv.

The nurse called me at work the other day. Liv fell on the stairs at school. I was trying to keep it together at work, hoping for the best, yet fearing she had hurt her back. I get so frightened of the prospect of her having to get surgery. I find myself becoming snappy and overreacting to the small things, "YOU DIDN'T HANG UP YOUR COAT AGAIN???? GO TO YOUR ROOM FOREVER!!! AND GIVE ME YOUR CELL PHONE, WHICH YOU'LL NEVER GET BACK!!!" Then Liv gets mad at me, and seems to forget her own worries.

We had the dreaded eight-month x-ray appointment. Strangely, Liv's curves didn't grow. Instead, the x-ray showed that both curves were compensating for each other at 39°. What an amazing way to start the New Year. At that appointment, Dr. Mermelstein suggested that Liv could start weaning off the brace four- to six-hours a day, with the hope of being out of it during the day in about a year. At this time, she was twelve and almost 5 feet 5 inches with a Risser 4.

Unfortunately, Jeff and I received surprising news about fellow Curvy Girl Deanna. After many months post-brace, we learned that Deanna's curve had progressed and she was now awaiting corrective surgery. One of Liv's great fears is that she will start weaning and her curves will instantly increase. She'll leave the brace off periodically, yet she'll know intuitively when she needs to put it back on. I think her body tells her when it is ready. Since this last appointment with Dr. Mermelstein, I have significantly mellowed out. I have started putting more trust and faith in Liv knowing what is right for her body.

Every afternoon and weekend, Liv's head is buried in a book. Every night she cries. She is still odd kid out. And if you cannot see it through her baggy clothes, her mask of makeup, and meticulously straightened hair, then maybe you see it in her shuffle or her guarded body language. Sure, some of it's from being a teenage girl, but sometimes it seems like all she has is her scoliosis. Guitar lessons start next week and creative writing this Saturday. She's at the gym twice a week and with the good chiropractor once a week.

Liv seems sad, depressed, and withdrawn. What would her life be like without wearing a brace? We checked into surgery but it would only be cosmetic at this point. What if she could wear cute shoes and cool tight clothes like the other girls? What if she could bend and twist and run as fast as the other kids? What if she wasn't so self-conscious? Would she negotiate the social terrain of middle school differently without this brace? How different would she be without her scoliosis anger? How much taller would she be without two curves in her spine?

Liv will not attend Curvy Girls meetings anymore, preferring not to deal with her scoliosis any longer. I guess maybe she feels that by ignoring it, she won't give it any power to lord over her. I also know that she feels like she doesn't fit in because some of the other girls are "done" with their journey, either through bracing, or with both bracing and surgery. I try to convince her to come with me, knowing that the journey is never really over. Leah has to live with rods in her back; Rachel still has to have her back checked, and poor Deanna, who thought she was finally "done," headed to surgery.

Liv and I return to Dr. Mermelstein in a month and a half for an exam. If he feels the curve has changed, he'll take an x-ray. She has been braced for two years now. I no longer fool myself that the rest of her time in the brace will be easy. I know the curves could increase, or she could need surgery.

I wear the white Curvy Girl necklace of "Hope" around my neck, on my chain of Lapis Lazuli, which wards off negative energy (very useful when one works with the public!). I hope that Liv will feel confident and comfortable in herself one day. Until that day comes, I will be her backbone. I will try to give her the support and courage she needs to embrace every day.

In the mornings, I help her put her boots on because she cannot bend. She has to take off the brace to brush and style her long hair, which she cannot reach otherwise. She cannot pick up a pencil from the floor during class, nor does she dare sneeze or cough, for fear of that loud Velcro® RRRRRRIIIIIIIPPPPPPPP of the straps. Sometimes, even the slightest movement causes the straps to pop. She is the only one sitting during chorus because she cannot stand for long periods in the brace. She is the last one in the locker room after gym and after-school sports, hiding the brace until everyone has gone. She shies from friendly hugs and phony air kisses in the school halls, so no one will feel the brace.

She feels different. She feels insecure. She finds temporary refuge in her books, writing, music, shopping, reality TV, rage, and tears.

WHAT I'VE LEARNED

There is nothing quite as devastating as seeing your child in pain, physical and/or emotional. When I get frustrated and start yelling about Liv's choosing not to practice her exercises, I forget the sickened, helpless feelings that I have when I see the scars under her arms, back, and hip. I forget how amazed and proud I am of her that she wore and dealt with the Boston Brace through her physical torment for months. I forget how in awe I am of her emotional strength when either of us is ready to give up. Liv keeps putting that brace back on. I forget that every day Liv goes to middle school and battles her self-consciousness to get through the day. I forget that I admire this child; I adore this child, and will continue to do whatever it takes to help this child heal her back, even if it means swallowing my pride and borrowing money to afford the "best" care. Even if it means remembering to shut my big mouth and let Liv cry, complain, and just be angry. I also now know that I have to speak up for my child and sometimes challenge the professionals. I cannot allow my daughter to go through any more than she has to. I've learned the hard way that being nice or submissive to a doctor because of their title is not helping my child. It is my role as her mother to speak up for her.

I made too many mistakes, including not being forceful enough with the original pediatric orthopedic surgeon to demand better care. Allowing some idiot x-ray technician to tell me that shielding Liv's ovaries was not possible, or not realizing that I have to provide the school district with documentation allowing Liv extra time after gym. When Liv was diagnosed, I had NO earthly idea about whom to talk to or what questions to ask.

> I also learned that
> "pediatric orthopedic surgeon"
> doesn't necessarily mean
> specializing in scoliosis.

The Internet gave too many options, the library not enough. It wasn't until I emailed JoEllen of the Scoliosis Association of Long Island, and she put me in touch with Leah and Robin, that my life had changed. There were other scoli-parents out there struggling with similar questions. It's not just me!

I still feel helpless and awful when I see Liv having a bad brace/ back day. But now I am better prepared to speak up for her at school and with the doctors.

And, once in a while, just for laughs for both Liv and me, on Liv's medical history forms where it asks if anyone else in the family has been diagnosed with scoliosis, I'll write . . . "The dog."

PART II
EMBRACING FASHION

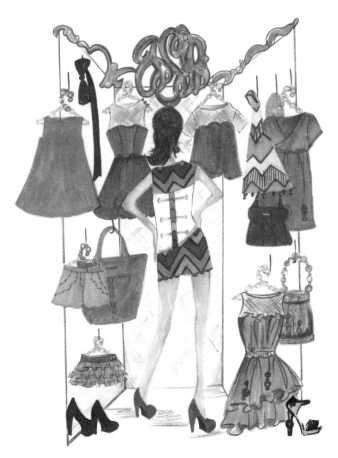

RACHEL MULVANEY
Long Island Curvy Girl Shopping Consultant

What to Shop For

As a teenage girl who wore a back brace throughout middle school, I understand the internal struggles you are going through. I know the fear you live with, whether it's going to the next doctor's appointment, taking a new x-ray, or dreading what others will think when they see your back brace. This section is designed to help each individual girl feel confident and beautiful in her brace.

BECOMING A FASHIONISTA

I personally believe the easiest seasons to shop for are winter and fall. There are so many different choices that will complement all figures. My Curvy Girl friends and I wish we had the variety of clothing options available now, when we were braced: oversized sweaters, scarves, leather/denim jackets, cardigans, knitted sweatshirts, off-the-shoulder baggy shirts, you name it! All of those things can easily become part of your exciting new wardrobe.

TRENDY TOPS FOR BRACING

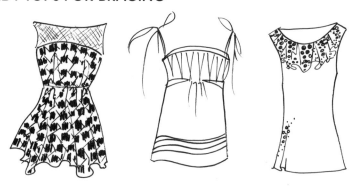

The seasons that girls fear most are spring and summer, however it's not as bad as you think. Sure you cannot wear those heavy/thick sweaters that hide your brace straps, but there are plenty of cute tops light enough to wear in the warmer weather that can still complement your outfit. Baby-doll flare-out shirts are the biggest hit during these seasons. They're loose and won't stick to you. Layering is key.

Materials such as nylon/spandex are great choices. Try to find camisoles that have no seams; they're more comfortable and they don't leave any imprints on your skin.

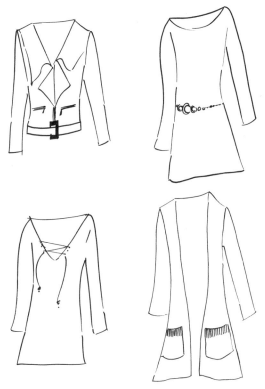

Fall and winter months are probably the easiest to dress for. Long sweaters and jackets best complement your brace. As you shop for clothes, remember to have fun and don't be afraid to experiment with what works best for you.

LEGGINGS, JEGGINGS AND MORE…

Jeggings are excellent jean replacements. You no longer need to buy jeans a size too big or feel uncomfortable tucking your denim under the brace. Jeggings are made with elastic material and they stretch to fit all types of figures. They're comfortable, affordable, and fashionable.

When choosing jeans, girls always contemplate the question, "What's more comfortable, wearing the jeans inside the brace, or going up a size and putting the bottoms over the brace?" It's a personal choice, but I was able to wear mine over my brace.

Sweatpants, gym shorts, and yoga pants also offer girls another option for comfort in the brace.

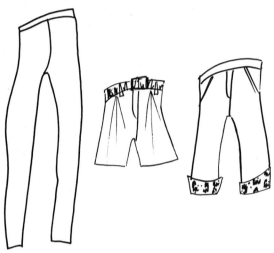

STYLISH SKIRTS

Skirts are extremely useful because they're easy to wear over your brace. The best kinds are the flare-out, ruffled ones. You should avoid pencil skirts because they're too tight and will show the bulkiness of your brace.

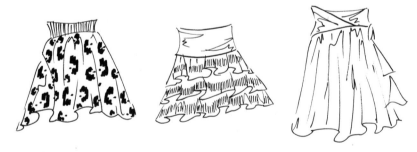

DRESSES

I know everyone wants to wear skin-tight clothes during the spring and summer seasons, but look at all the great fashionable options you have! While shopping for dresses, avoid any material that is thin and clingy, as these will only put an emphasis on your brace straps. Try looking for items that have a flare or baggier style.

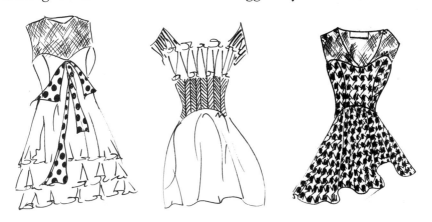

Accessorizing

SCARVES AND BELTS

In consideration of girls whose back brace has a shoulder strap, scarves are perfect!

Here are some examples:

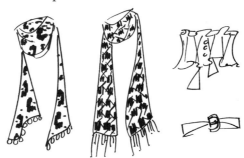

And finally, another accessory that can complement your outfit while in your brace is a belt. It can be used as a distraction from the brace. People will be drawn to the belt, not the brace.

PUTTING IT ALL TOGETHER

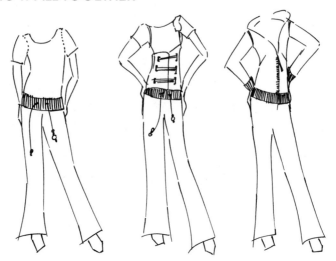

Using sweatpants and jackets is probably the easiest trick to fool people from knowing you have a back brace on. Remember, zip-up jackets can be interchangeable with many other bottoms.

The Curvy Girls of Chicago launched a brace-friendly clothing line—Hope's Closet, www.hopescloset.com. We invite you to explore the site and share your fashion ideas with Hope.

PART III

TAKING CHARGE

A Conversation for Teens with
Curvy Girls Leah & Rachel

A Message from Leah

I didn't ask for scoliosis; it just happened. You didn't ask to wear a plastic form-fitting back brace, but here it is.

We don't have control over certain things that happen in our lives. As kids, we have even less control, which is why it's so important to be able to have a voice in your medical care.

The first thing I want you to know is that there is no such thing as being too young to understand what is being done to you. While in the doctor's office, even for just a regular check-up, please make your voice heard. If there's something on your mind, ask. Make sure the doctors don't just talk to your parents—but that they talk to you as well!

This is YOUR body and you NEED to know what is going on. Knowing what's happening makes the process so much easier and less stressful. When your parents see that you're comfortable, they will feel a little more at ease as well.

Give voice to your thoughts and opinions. When you are going through something tough like we are, you need to express yourself.

We need to speak with passion about how to deal with and overcome our problems. I think a lot of us hold back. We quiet our own opinions or ideas because we're scared of what others may think.

Don't let someone quiet your heart.

Leah

A Message from Rachel

If you're like Leah and I, you probably still remember the first time you saw "it."

I cried.

Leah cried, too.

We had no idea how we were going to wear a brace for a minute, let alone for hours, days …years.

We know firsthand that going through this journey alone only makes it harder. Let us help you along the way. We've been there, and we know what you're going through.

We'll tell you everything you need to know about bracing, and answer all those questions you were too intimidated to ask your doctor or orthotist. We want you to know that the pain and suffering of being alone ends today.

Rachel

A Brace ... Are They Crazy?

Why do we have to wear a back brace?

From two girls who have been braced for years, let us tell you why bracing is important. The brace is designed to help maintain and control the progression of your curves. If we don't wear our brace, the curves will more than likely progress. Our biggest growth spurts occur during our adolescent years. For someone with scoliosis, this is also the time when our curves progress the most. Remember the brace is actually supporting your body in a more balanced position, which is why the brace initially feels so uncomfortable.

What does it feel like to wear a back brace?

We like to compare adjusting to a back brace to getting used to orthodontic braces. Remember that restricted, tight feeling on your teeth when they were first put on? Remember how sore your mouth was until your teeth adjusted to the hardware? And yet a week later, you were back to eating whatever you wanted. That same reaction will occur with your back brace. The more you wear it, the easier it will get.

Does it hurt to wear a back brace?

It's uncomfortable at first to wear the back brace. For some, it might actually feel a little painful because your body is used to being pulled towards the dominant curve side, and the brace is trying to change that. Your body feels weird because it's actually being put into alignment for the first time. Again, it will get better the more you wear the brace.

How tight does the brace have to be?

Did you ever see a person wear loose braces on their teeth? Well the same rule applies to our back braces. In order for our back brace to be doing its job, it should be worn snug/tight. Your hands should not be able to slip down into your brace. However, initially you don't want to wear it too tight—that will make your adjustment to bracing more difficult. Your best bet is to ask your orthotist to put a mark on your straps to indicate the ideal position to where the straps should be tightened.

How will I know the difference between what is considered normal discomfort and pain that I should tell my parent or doctor about?

Some tenderness is normal. Remember, the brace is trying to resist the natural curve of your body. But if your skin begins to bruise, redness doesn't go away, your skin begins to bleed, or you feel sharp pains going down your leg or around your abdomen, it's time to tell your parent and orthotist. None of these symptoms are acceptable because bracing should not be causing significant pain or bruising. Your parents need to contact your orthotist to find out what is causing the problem.

Do I have to wear the brace every day? Is it bad if sometimes I cheat a little?

Yes. Brace compliance is very important. And yes, you can cheat, but try to make up for the hours out of the brace. The bottom line is that you're only hurting yourself by not complying with the hours that your doctor has set. Always ask yourself, "Is this worth it?" You don't want to regret your decision years down the road. And remember, if we took off our orthodontic braces whenever we wanted to, our teeth would never have good results.

What is the best undershirt or tee shirt you can recommend to wear under my brace?

Most girls like the non-ribbed, cotton boy's sleeveless undershirts. Wearing this shirt under your brace adds comfort and prevents the skin from having direct contact with the brace.

Is there anything I can do to prepare my skin?

Yes. Applying a little witch hazel around your abdomen will help to toughen your skin. We have also noticed that applying Gold Bond Medicated Body Powder® under your tee shirt helps to prevent abrasions from the brace.

I sometimes feel sharp edges around my brace. What causes this?

If the sharp edges are from the padding wearing down, congratulations, this means that you are consistently wearing your brace! Once again, let your parents know what is going on. They will need to make an appointment with the orthotist. More than likely the orthotist

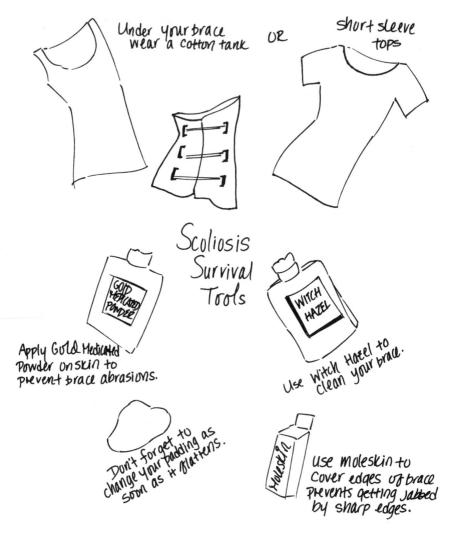

Under your brace wear a cotton tank

OR

short sleeve tops

Scoliosis Survival Tools

Apply Gold Medicated Powder on skin to prevent brace abrasions.

Use Witch Hazel to clean your brace.

Don't forget to change your padding as soon as it flattens.

Use moleskin to cover edges of brace. Prevents getting jabbed by sharp edges.

will need to add some padding around the edges of your brace. In the meantime, purchase some moleskin at a local pharmacy. Have your parents cut and place the moleskin in the areas that are sharp until you are able to have your orthotist make the necessary adjustments.

What can be done about the holes in my shirts from the metal on the brace?
Haven't we told you about shopping for new clothes?! You will need to go shopping to buy clothes that work best with your brace. When you shop for clothes, make sure to choose sturdy material. Also, put

moleskin over the metal parts of the brace. Be prepared to replace the moleskin periodically because it will fall off.

How can I keep my brace clean?
We wiped our braces down with household cleansers like Fantastik® and Formula 409®.

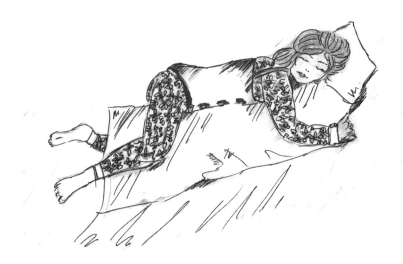

How can you sleep with a back brace?
Leah shared this tip during one of our first support group meetings. Her trick was to put a pillow or two in between her legs to balance out the unevenness in our hips. This little trick may help you get a better night's sleep. Another great tip is to purchase a foam mattress pad topper, the more padding the better for extra support and comfort.

I'm nervous my friends will find out I am wearing a back brace. Any advice on what to do?
Yes. Tell your friends. We know you're scared; we have all been there. Keeping it a secret makes it worse. It will be so much easier on you to tell them the truth. You will be surprised how supportive they can be. They will probably have a ton of questions for you, but this is because they don't understand what you are going through. Honestly and patiently explain to them what scoliosis is and what the brace is doing. This will help them understand and better support you.

Can I wear my brace during activities?

That depends on the activity. Your back brace is not worn for bike riding, running, participating in gym class, dance classes, or other sports, and certainly not swimming. Doing these activities while wearing your brace could actually hurt you. If you are not sure whether or not you should wear your back brace, it's always best to ask your doctor.

Do I have to shower with my brace on?

No. You don't shower with your brace on.

Is it normal to have bruises from my brace?

Absolutely NOT. If you are bruising, tell your parents.

How long does it take to get used to wearing the brace?

A well-made brace should take about a week to get used to.

How many hours do I have to wear this brace?

That will depend on your orthopedic doctor. Leah wore her brace for twenty-two hours a day, while Rachel's orthopedic doctor instructed her to wear it for sixteen hours.

Will I ever like wearing my brace?

That's up to you. As much as you'll dislike your back brace in the beginning, it'll be easier on you if you change your feelings about your brace. Always remember that your back brace is there for a reason. It's protecting you by fighting against the curves in your spine. Maintaining a positive mental attitude, "I will get through this," will help make life easier.

School Nurse Letter

After listening to Curvy Girls talk about the difficulty they have with bracing in school, my parents and I put together a letter that Curvy Girls can give to school nurses to help them understand what we are going through and how important their role is in our lives. You may want to use this letter at your school.

Visit www.straighttalkscoliosis.com to download a copy.

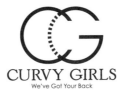

CURVY GIRLS
We've Got Your Back

International Scoliosis Support Groups
Leah Stoltz, Founder 2006
www.curvygirlsscoliosis.com

Dear School Nurse,

This letter is to share with you my experience having scoliosis, and how you can help other affected students deal with their everyday challenges.

When I was diagnosed and endured three years of bracing and, ultimately, major spine surgery, it was my School Nurse and Physical Education teacher who made a tremendous difference in my school adjustment. My School Nurse's office was a safe place to remove my brace and store it during gym glass. She reassured me that I could ask her for assistance at any time; I felt that she was very sensitive toward my condition.

It's very important to realize that, aside from being a medical condition, scoliosis affects us most emotionally. Kids in middle school try very hard to feel like they fit in. Wearing this uncomfortable contraption to school every day poses some very embarrassing situations that can become more traumatic than most people realize. Oftentimes, kids with scoliosis try very hard to keep their disease a secret from peers, which can result in emotional stress.

Kids with scoliosis frequently face challenges such as:
* *Acute self-consciousness around body image and braces*

- *Avoidance of situations (i.e., gym class, swimming pools, school dances, and proms) where the secret of the brace or body deformity might be exposed*
- *Fears of facing major spine surgery*

Students with scoliosis need to feel that they have an ally in the school. You can help the student with their adjustment in many ways such as:

1. *Ensure that they have a person to seek out, and a private space where they can remove, hide, or store their brace, so that they can avoid questions from their peers;*
2. *Communicate the student's needs and concerns to other school personnel, such as late passes and additional set of textbooks (to reduce carrying a heavy load);*
3. *Make sure that scoliosis is discussed in health classes; and*
4. *Connect the student with counseling services if they show signs of anxiety or depression.*

It's very important that the school be sensitive to children who are being braced for scoliosis and possibly facing surgery. Your acceptance and attitude towards your student can make a world of difference. I know, because they made a difference for me!

Thank you for your consideration.

Sincerely,

Leah Stoltz, Founder

In an effort to help young people understand more about scoliosis and know what to expect at a screening, the National Scoliosis Foundation (www.scoliosis.org) created a ten-minute scoliosis screening video, "Catch the Curve." NSF and a Curvy Girl are available to attend a pre-screening session to discuss the video and tell their own story.

Bone Nutrition Trivia

If you have scoliosis, you can't afford to compromise the health of your bones any further. You need to be especially mindful of avoiding products that deplete your supply of calcium.

Robyn Rexford, R.D. and Nutritionist shares some interesting facts with the Curvy Girls:

Did you know?
Caffeine, an ingredient in soda, depletes calcium, which then weakens our bones.

Caffeine depletes bone density. To reduce the risk of osteoporosis later in life, it is crucial that females in their teens and twenties build up bone mass.

If you are anticipating spinal fusion surgery, it is most important to make sure that your bones are in the best shape possible.

Did you know?
Milk contains calcium to build bones. The only significant difference between skim and whole milk is FAT content. The difference in calcium content is negligible. So, the only thing you get more of by drinking whole milk is fat.

Did you know?
The best drink you can have is water-water-water—or low-fat milk!

Did you know?
One of the main ingredients in cola is phosphoric acid.

Did you know?
Dark soda (cola) can clean your porcelain toilet, remove corrosion off of car battery terminals, and clean blood from accident scenes. And yet, this is what we drink!

How to Prepare for Surgery

BEFORE THE BIG DAY

Nutrition: Getting your body into the best possible condition will help in your recovery process. Eating balanced meals creates a healthy body to promote healing. Antioxidant rich foods such as berries can aid in the healing process. Papaya and kiwis are rich in zinc, which helps build your immune system. Don't forget to drink plenty of water leading up to and after surgery in order to cleanse your body.

You will want to limit the intake of synthetic sugar (especially high fructose corn syrup), because the excess intake of sugar affects our immune system.

No ibuprofen (Motrin®, Advil®, certain menstrual pain medications) for three- to six-months prior to fusion surgery and up until your physician says your spine is fully fused. Because ibuprofen interferes with blood clotting, it can interfere with the fusion process. So it's important to check with your surgeon's office before taking prescribed or over-the-counter medication, or any type of herbal supplements.

The Logroll: Practice makes perfect!

Have you ever rolled down a hill sideways for fun? This is called a "logroll" and is just what you need to be able to do after surgery to help you get out of bed. (Well, not the rolling down the hill part!) While at home practice turning from your back to your side as if you were a log. This means keeping your body stiff like a wood log, while turning your whole body as one unit from your back to your side. No body part turns without the other parts. By maintaining equal distribution from your feet to your head, you will not be using back muscles to turn. Whenever you change positions, tighten your abdominal muscles.

An easy way to tighten ab muscles is by taking a breath in and then slowly letting it out while pulling your belly button in toward your spine. Practice this when getting out of bed each morning, and it will be easier to do after surgery.

After you have rolled onto your side, slowly scoot to the edge of the bed and put your legs over the edge. Use your arms to support yourself, while sitting up.

So let's strengthen your arm muscles, and while you're at it, how about those thigh muscles to help you on and off chairs and ... the toilet too!

Core strengthening exercises are good for everyone but will especially help you with your post-surgery movement. The stronger your stomach muscles, the less stress on your back muscles.

Leah's Surgery Tips

- Know what is best for YOU and make people aware of it.

- Need to be distracted the night before? Ask your parents to have a sleepover with your best friend.

- You'll want your hair away from your face, or pulled back, because you won't be able to wash it for a few days. I know a couple of girls who had their hair cut dramatically short in order to avoid dealing with it during recovery. Curvy Girl Rachel and her older sister came over the night before surgery to French braid my hair and give me a facial to help relax me. The braid kept my hair in place.

- If you wear glasses, make sure you're happy with them. There's no way you're going to want to put your contacts in. (The pictures of me in those horrible wire-rimmed glasses are quite embarrassing!)

- Don't bother buying new sleepwear. Believe it or not, you will be relieved that you are just wearing one of those "lovely" open-back hospital gowns that allow easy access. You don't want to pull anything over your head because it's difficult to raise your arms up. Just make sure someone holds your gown closed when you are walking the halls or put on sweatpants. Remember, no mooning!

- You may want to pack your own pillow, fuzzy blanket, large sweats or oversized tee shirt, slippers, iPod with headphones, cell phone and charger, and anything that helps you relax. I brought a laptop.

- Some girls want to have friends and family visit them in the hospital, and some are against it. Make sure that you verbalize your desire to your parents and other people. This is YOUR recovery time and you need to be as comfortable as possible. You don't want to be feeling miserable in the hospital, and on top of that, start feeling worse when you hear that your cute family friend who you've had a crush on since you were five is coming to visit. Personally, I loved having people visit, even though I was embarrassed beyond belief with how

I looked. They helped me take my mind off of things and broke the monotony of seeing only the nurses, my parents, and my brother.

- Having a positive mental attitude is important going into surgery. Positive thoughts help to accelerate the healing process. Focus on something that you are going to get from having surgery. Yes, it can even be that new iPod. Only 5 feet 1 inch, I was excited about being taller, and couldn't wait to stand up next to my 5-foot-2-inch mom to see my new height. So much so, that the next morning after surgery, I insisted that the nurse help me to stand. When I leaned up against my mom, with the nurse's support, I started to cry ... sure enough I was looking down at her!

   My mom reminded me that while I may be taller, she was still in charge!

- **Surprise! Surprise!** What is the **one thing** you hope doesn't happen the day you are finally ready to go for surgery? Even if you are not expecting to get your period during your time in the hospital— EXPECT IT! And that's exactly what happened to me. I couldn't believe it when I got my period the night before my surgery. Beth Roach, my friend and pediatric intensive care nurse says, "I know it seems like a cruel joke but probably 75 percent of girls will get their period. This is possibly your body's response to the stress of going for surgery. You may want to pack your preferred products, unless you enjoy the huge OB pads that most hospitals supply."

- You know how adults say that we are the ADD generation because we just can't focus on one thing at a time? Well, multiply that by twenty. I had NO attention span to read books or the magazines people brought me (and I love to read). I mostly just flipped through the magazines to see the pictures and watched TV. I couldn't concentrate, which was probably a factor of the anesthesia. I did, however, put the laptop on my chest the first chance I could, which was the next day after surgery. Mom says I fell asleep instant messaging. Who remembers "instant messaging?"

- Oh yeah, don't be frightened when you do see your face. My eyes and face were pretty puffy from being face down for so long during surgery.

- One of our biggest fears is about pain after surgery. Nurse Beth said it best, *"Pain is to be managed."* That is done with oral medication and a medicine pump. You will repeatedly be asked for your "pain number." This is a 1-10 scale: 0 being pain-free and 10 being the worst. You need to say something right away if you are in pain.

- You will be given a medicine pump after surgery, so don't be afraid to use it! The pump is programmed to only give safe doses of medication based on your weight. You CANNOT overdose and will not become addicted in such a short period of time. So press the button when you feel the slightest pain.

- Press a small pillow over your stomach to support you when you cough or sneeze.

- Don't sit on a soft chair or couch; it's too difficult to get up!

- So you want to go home? You get to go home when your pain is under control, when you can walk around, manage stairs and eat regular food. Warning: Use the toilet before you go home. Constipation can occur because of reduced food and fluid intake, so make sure to drink plenty of water. If you are constipated, ask the nurse for a stool softener. You don't want to be straining. Remember: Be kind to those back muscles!

- Our badge of honor! We don't want to hide our scars. Now we have something on the outside to show what we've been through on the inside. Our scars are like our battle wounds.

- Protect your scar. Protect the incision and the area around it from the sun, either by keeping the area covered or by applying a sunblock when you go outside. Continue to do so for a full year. These efforts won't make your scar disappear but they will facilitate the healing process. Remember, too, that sunscreens should never be used on open stitches, so wait until your surgeon gives you the go ahead.

- Last, but not least, it's important to have a good relationship with your surgeon. I was lucky to have a great relationship with my doctor. One of the best memories I have is of waking up the morning after surgery to the touch of my doctor's hand and his gentle voice saying my name. I looked up and there he was.

Rachel's Journey to Scoliosis Rehab
Rachel Mulvaney, age 15

After almost two years being out of my brace, my curve progressed from 35° to 42°. The research for writing this book educated us on a European-based treatment called the Schroth Method. This method uses specific exercises that might reverse or stop my curve from progressing. On August 15th, 2010, my mom and I flew to the Scoliosis Rehab facility in Wisconsin for two weeks of training so I could learn these exercises. I posted my experience on the Curvy Girls website for everyone to follow. This is my journey.

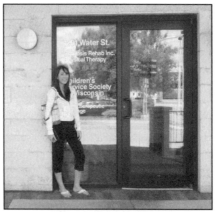

Rachel at Scoliosis Rehab

DAY 1

Don't let the smile fool you; I was quite nervous before I walked through these doors. Once I did, I was greeted by the most dedicated and passionate group of people.

My first day started off with a review about myself, what activities I like to do, and generally getting a little history on my scoliosis. Due to the fact that every curve is different, it is important for the physical therapists to know what type of activities we do. By learning this information, they are able to correct and suggest an alternative way to do our activities without our bodies collapsing into our curves.

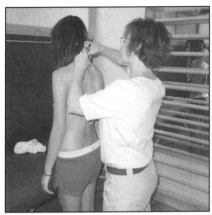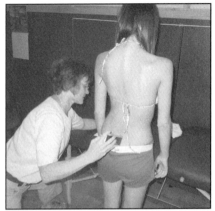

First day at Scoliosis Rehab

Beth Janssen (above) takes my measurements and later tests my strength and flexibility. Later on, Beth reviews my x-rays and we learn that I have three curves, not two, which means I now need to learn five steps to keep my body in alignment.

I ended the first day by learning a new breathing technique, which is what I am doing in the photo below.

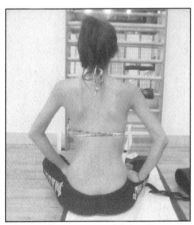

Elongating pose and Schroth pose

DAY 2

Hey everyone, day two in rehab, and I thought I should share some information I learned today. If you get muscle spasms, this will explain it all!

Since scoliosis forces our curves to grow towards one side more than the other, it causes the muscles in our backs to be in an imbalanced position. The curvature development and rotational pull of the spine will lead to collapsed areas and unevenness in our bodies. The muscles on the concave (curving inward) side are shortened, and on the convex (curving outward, bulging) part of the back, the muscles are stretched out and elongated. Due to the muscles having different resting lengths, they cannot have equal activation; therefore, it can create back pain and muscle spasms. So what we worked on today was learning how to shift my body into a position that decreased the pressure on my muscles that are close to my large curve.

DAYS 3 & 4

Today was the first day that I was able to walk in alignment. It felt weird ... but it was a great feeling to see that when I looked in the mirror, I was straight for the first time!

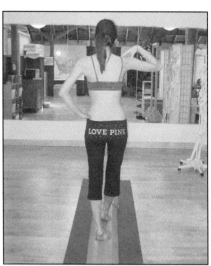

Schroth walk

By the third day, the amount of change I see in my body is crazy. I feel myself getting stronger and can feel the difference from within.

One of the exercises I am currently doing is training my breathing. We're working on expanding the concave side of my rib cage where the collapse of my curve is. By breathing into my weak spot and my weak side, it literally puts my spine in a straight position. It's like how we all try to disguise our braces by layering clothes and hiding it. Well, by me doing these exercises consistently, it will permanently disguise the appearance of my scoliosis.

Here I am working on how to grow taller, which is called "elongate."

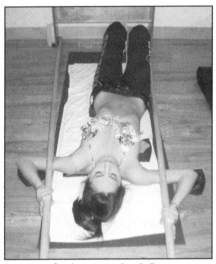

Supine - growing taller

One technique of elongating is by using straps to put on my waist, which we then attach to a bar. I lay on the floor with a small beanbag under my left hip, one under my right rib cage/shoulder blade, and another under my left shoulder. We use these to untwist the rotation. I continue to breathe deeply. As I do so, I'm using the muscles in my ribs to grow taller and taller with each breath. Along with this, I'm expanding my right rib cage, which will symmetrically balance my rib cages. I literally feel my spine being pulled straight just by my own breaths!

DAY 5

On Friday I begin to do the exercises more independently. Instead of having my physical therapists Beth or Patti Orthwein help me elongate, I can do it on my own. I'm becoming more aware of where my body is in space. In other words, when I'm not doing my exercises and my body is no longer in the correct position, I've noticed that I collapse into my curve way too much. We have habits like slouching and not sitting in good posture throughout our lives, and it's hard to break these bad habits. However, little do we know that when we have scoliosis and we slouch, we're doing much more than just collapsing into our curves; we're also causing damage to the discs in our backs. How are they becoming damaged? Well, when we slouch, it puts pressure on the discs. When these discs are completely squished it's called a "herniated disc" and pain will be consistent. One of the best things about this clinic is how much education you receive. I am taught all about the development of my curves, what causes my pain, and now, what I can do to prevent it.

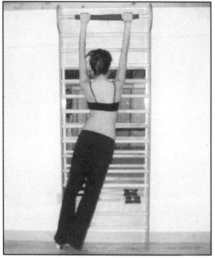

Pendulum

The more I work on doing these exercises, the better I get at it. This above exercise is called "Pendulum," where I go on the top bar and swing. On the first day I was capable of only doing four or five. Now I'm up to thirty on day five. I can breathe longer and elongate better too! Monday, I'll be working on doing more exercises on my own, so I'll let you all know how that goes. I am so surprised about how much I'm able to do. I'm doing things that I never thought I was capable of doing because I was always in pain.

DAYS 6 & 7

I'll be combining both day six and seven because I haven't necessarily done anything new. The difference between this week and last week is that this week I'm doing everything more independently. I now know how to put my body in alignment, as well as perform the exercises on my own with very few corrections from the therapist. I am slowly beginning to see all the changes that my body is doing. One of the things that stood out the most in this journey occurred on day six.

I was doing this exercise called "Side Laying." The position for that is laying on my left side with a cushion under my left hip, left shoulder, and a pad for my head. As I breathe deeply, I try to open up the weak side (left rib cage), weak spot (under my right rib cage), and push my right rib cage forward. While I was doing that, I heard my mom and Beth in awe from the results. Feeling frustrated because I couldn't internally feel what they were physically seeing, Beth ran her fingers down each vertebrae of my spine. For my whole life, all I ever experienced when my doctor examined my spine was his hands swirling in different directions. However, today for the first time, someone's hands went down my back in a straight line. A mirror was put in position and I was able to not only see what they did, but feel it too. It was a great day!

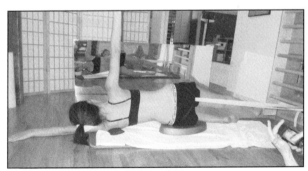
Side Laying

DAYS 8 & 9

I cannot believe my time here is coming to an end, and to be honest, I am shocked that it went so fast. Once again I chose to combine two days, since a lot of this time is now perfecting what I've already been taught.

On Wednesday, I was taught something new—the proper way to work out my abdominals. First Beth asked me to show her how I normally would exercise my abs. Excitedly, I laid on the ground and proceeded to demonstrate my favorite double leg lifts. For those of you who aren't sure what this exercise is, allow me to explain. You lie on the ground and swiftly raise your legs up in a 45° angle. You then slowly bring your legs down as low as you can and then split them apart, bring them back together, hold them for a few seconds (or as long as you can), bring your legs back up to that 45° angle, and then repeat the pattern about twenty-five times.

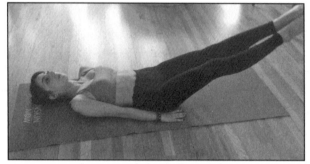

Improper abdominal excercise

After one performance of this exercise, Beth looked at me and asked, "Who taught you this exercise?" I told her that it was part of my warm-up exercises when I was taking dance for nine years. She then asked me never to do them again and explained how much damage I was doing to the already pressured discs in my spine. I would later learn that by doing double leg lifts, you're not giving your back the support it needs. The main problem when doing these leg lifts is that your back arches too much (increasing your lordosis), which would make it very difficult to maintain your pelvic corrections.

Beth then promised that the exercises she would be giving me would not only be safe for my spine, but would create the six-pack abs of my dreams.

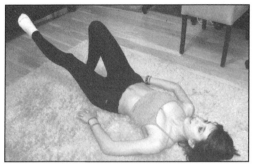

Correct abdominal excercise

By keeping one foot bent on the floor and the other raised, I am able to keep my back in a more stabilized position. Just as we would do in our normal pelvic correction, you give yourself slight lordosis and from that position you are able to control the way your hips shift. Also, when using one leg at a time, you're not increasing the rotation in your spine, something that is essential to avoid for someone with scoliosis.

After one afternoon of doing these "new and improved" ab exercises, my stomach felt like a rock. And the best part is they are actually easier than the ones I learned years ago in my dance classes.

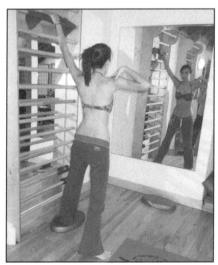

St. Andrews cross

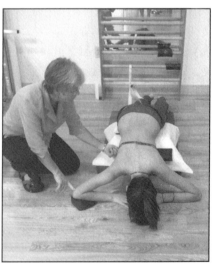

Patti assisting Prone on stool

On day nine, I was doing the exercises independently with either Beth or Patti correcting me only if it was needed. Before I left this afternoon, Beth gave me a book with a typed-up description of every exercise I've learned in the past two weeks, along with a picture of me doing the exercise as a reminder of what my body has to look like while doing them. I have nearly perfected each task and I am eager to say that I will be returning here next year to challenge myself and get new exercises to work on.

I truly hope one day soon that the Schroth Method will change the way doctors view scoliosis in this country. In my opinion, the Schroth Method exercises should be one of the first things offered to a child and her parents. I understand that this is a lifestyle change that some of us will need to do forever, but trust me when I say, "It's worth it."

As a teenager, when we hear the word "forever," we either don't know what to expect, or freak out due to the thought of how big the time span is. I was told that within a month or two these exercises would be easier for me. Well, I'm on week two and I've already adapted to these changes. I came here suffering with pain nearly every day for five years, and now the only time I truly have pain is when my body is out of neutral, meaning my pelvis is out of balance and rotated.

LAST DAY AT THE SCOLIOSIS REHAB

Coming here two weeks ago, I was both skeptical and nervous. Being the first one in our support group to try this type of treatment, I was excited but still scared. I worried about whether these exercises would really help me, would I be able to do the exercises, and mostly, would I continue to do them? I told my mom that I owe the girls in our support group my honest feelings about this experience here at Scoliosis Rehab. Learning these exercises was a lot of hard work, but it was not harder than learning to adapt to wearing a back brace for sixteen hours a day for nearly three years.

Are the exercises the same for all of us that have scoliosis? No. Just like the fact that no curves are the same, not everyone will have the same exercise program. The Schroth Method is about providing you with tools to help your scoliosis. Can the Schroth Method guarantee to stop the progression of scoliosis? No. There will always be curves that progress no matter what preventions we take, however, learning these exercises will never be a waste of time for a scoliotic person.

I've been in everyone's shoes with regard to bracing and doctor visits every four- to six-months. Each visit, when I'd go in for my x-rays (just like you guys do today), the doctor would examine my back and I'd literally hold my breath until he would announce whether my curve progressed or not. It was the worst feeling in the world, feeling this helpless, even though I did everything I was asked to do. But after nearly five years, I don't have to feel this pressure or the frustration of feeling powerless. For the first time since I was eleven and put into a back brace, I feel like I have taken back what I had lost—control over my own body. For five years, I complained to many doctors about back, shoulder, and hip pain, and no one truly believed me, but these therapists understood my pain.

After three days of being here, my pain was getting less and less. Today, I'm leaving totally pain free thanks to the invaluable lessons I've learned. My only real regret is wishing I had known about this method of exercise while my spine was still growing.

I will leave Scoliosis Rehab with a videotape of myself performing each exercise. Beth will do a voice-over on the tape, reinforcing what I need to be striving for in order to execute each position to the highest benefit for my body. My goal is to be able to do each position well and be able to maintain this position for about five minutes. This isn't such a terrible goal to strive for, especially if you're doing these exercises with your iPod in your ear. I have absolutely no regrets of giving up two weeks of my summer vacation and coming to the Scoliosis Rehab. The tools I have learned, I hope to carry with me for the rest of my life. Again, was it hard work? Yes, but now ask me, "Was it worth it?" Absolutely! Now you decide. Look at my results.

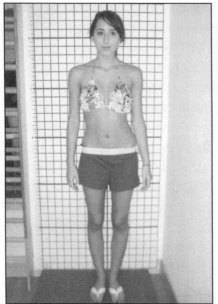
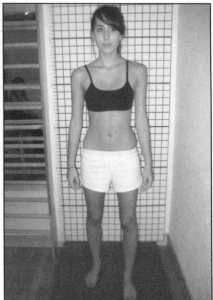

First day at the Scoliosis Rehab   Two weeks later

As you can see my shoulders are level, my hips are more centered, and my overall posture is entirely different than it was when I entered the program. Notice my right foot slightly behind my left foot. This change allows me to even out my hips which gave me my new postural position.

AFTER SCOLIOSIS REHAB—AGE 16

Four months later, I had my first follow-up visit with my orthopedic doctor since going to the Scoliosis Rehab clinic. For the first time in five years, I was not in pain. After a brief conversation regarding my experiences at the Scoliosis Rehab, Dr. Labiak began my examination. I stood up, bent forward, and he placed the Scoliometer on my back. As he wrote down the information in my chart, my mom asked if he noticed a change. He smiled and said, "Yes. If Rachel were to have a scoliosis school screening tomorrow, she would pass."

"What does that mean?" my mother asked.

He explained, "When the kids go in for their school screening exams, a Scoliometer reading of 5 to 7 is considered within normal range; Rachel is now a 7!" He reminded me that this does not necessarily mean that the measurement of my curve (Cobb angle) is different. "That is something we won't know until your x-rays in five months." By then, it would have been a year since my last x-rays were taken and I would have been doing the Schroth Method for eight full months. As an added bonus, we found an old orthopedic evaluation form dated two years prior showing a Scoliometer exam score of my ATR (angle of trunk rotation) and it was a 15. That's quite a difference! Sure felt like Christmas came early.

Five months later, we returned to take new x-rays. As we waited anxiously to find out if the exercises had helped to hold my curve from progressing, Dr. Labiak began to mark and measure my curves on the x-rays. It seemed like forever, and then he finally announced that my thoracic curve was 30°! I was shocked and wanted to scream, but knew this wasn't the place. My curve decreased 12°! My lumbar curve went from 26° to 22°! I think Dr. Labiak was as shocked as we were. He continued to compare both x-rays and concluded that technically this shouldn't have happened to a child who has been skeletally mature for two and a half years. Dr. Labiak was very happy for me. I just hope that he will tell his other patients about this treatment.

The reduction in my curves fuels me to continue exercising five days a week, twenty- to thirty-minutes a day. My new posture has become second nature. The point of doing the exercises is to make the muscles strong enough to maintain "correction" all the time. It's like having an internal brace. Sometimes I chuckle to myself when I am asked when I had surgery. But it frustrates me when I hear that my corrections are not accurate because I stood in my pelvic corrections for my x-rays. Why wouldn't I when I hold my body this way all the time? So when my x-rays are taken, or when I'm sitting, walking or standing, I remain in that same position—neutral.

These exercises have changed my life and I am excited to share my experiences with other families. My future goal is to continue to raise awareness about the positive effects the Schroth Method offers, a method that eliminated my back pain and prevented me from needing spinal fusion surgery.

PART IV
PARENT SUPPORT

Five Stages of Coping with Scoliosis

Kübler Ross' Five Stages of Coping with Grief provides a framework for understanding the process of how children, parents, and families cope with and adapt to scoliosis. Stages of coping are fluid, meaning that not everyone will start at the same place, nor experience all the stages, let alone proceed through them in a linear way. Instead, over the course of time, we may see children and parents exhibit features of all stages. The five stages in relation to scoliosis are:

Denial

This is the initial reaction we may have when first learning bad news. Pre-teens/teens diagnosed with scoliosis often do not want to acknowledge its existence. Kids who present with denial tend to be ashamed of having scoliosis. They may try to deny the unevenness of their body, avoid treatment, particularly bracing, while minimizing the risks of scoliosis.

Anger

Newly diagnosed children will often wonder, "Why me?" reflecting a sense of injustice as to why this disorder is happening to them. Anger can be displayed in increased arguments with parents over bracing compliance, as well as non-scoliosis issues.

Bargaining

"Let's Make a Deal." Active negotiations may ensue around how long, how often, whether, when, and when not they can wear their brace, participate in an exercise regime, or other recommended treatments. The effect of these negotiations is that the responsibility for decision-making falls squarely onto parents. At this stage, often because of a child's bargaining, families may seek out alternative treatments in a desperate attempt to have their child comply with treatment. The risk at this juncture is in being vulnerable to treatments that may not really be helpful and can result in losing precious time to employ more evidence-based approaches.

Depression

When efforts at bargaining prove futile, often after being confronted with curve progression as evidenced by a new set of x-rays and measurements, a feeling of sadness and resignation may start to set in. The child may begin to withdraw and isolate from peer contact and even from activities that they tend to enjoy, and sometimes appear to be walking around "in a fog." In response to bracing or more appointments for treatment, children in this stage might say, "I'm going to have surgery anyway, so why bother."

Acceptance

This is the stage of coming to terms with a scoliosis diagnosis, as well as recommended treatment(s). In this stage, children accept the reality that they have a condition that makes them different from other children, and which needs to be attended to in a way dictated by physicians and medical practitioners. It is a concession of power, realizing that the innocence of a "normal" body is physically gone and recognizing that this new reality of a spinal curvature with a treatment regimen is the current reality. It does not mean that the child is "okay" with having scoliosis, but they are now accepting of this new reality.

TEEN RESPONSE

Our children will use these various modes of coping when dealing with the challenges of scoliosis and wearing a brace. Some common scenarios and their corresponding coping stages are:

Refusers: (denial, anger, depression) don't want to have anything to do with scoliosis or brace treatment;

Pretenders: (denial, anger, depression) feign compliance, such as wearing the brace to school and then hiding it in their locker;

Negotiators: (denial, anger, bargaining) place the responsibility onto parent(s) of how long, how often, when and when not to wear the brace or exercise; often bargaining with parents;

Hiders: (anger, depression, acceptance) dutifully wear their brace and hope no one notices;

Accepters: (acceptance) compliant with brace wear and all recommended interventions, speak openly about their scoliosis.

Parents generally contact us when their child is either in the denial or depression stage and they are seeking help to get their child to agree to either follow through with bracing or, at least, feel better about their plight. In contrast, the girls that contact us directly are usually nearing the acceptance stage, but want guidance and affirmation from other girls in navigating the experience of scoliosis. The Curvy Girls support group experience enhances both acceptance and treatment compliance.

PARENT RESPONSE

Parents exhibit their own course of coping with the traumatic news of their child's newly diagnosed condition:

Denial and Isolation of Feelings

While some parents are not familiar with the signs and symptoms of scoliosis, once diagnosed, other parents might ignore or minimize their child's scoliosis due to fear of the unknown.

Some parents may readily accept the diagnosis of scoliosis and the required regimen of treatment, but minimize any emotional impact it has upon their child. Some of the parents in this phase go on "auto pilot," methodically isolating feelings, while concentrating on what needs to be done and not allowing emotions to take control. The "things to do" agenda prevails and dictates the plan for adapting to life with scoliosis.

Anger

Parents in this stage tend toward self-blame. They feel angry and guilty because this happened to their child under their watch. There's a sense of having failed parental duty, "I'm the parent. My job is to protect my child. Where did I go wrong? Why didn't I see the signs of this sooner?"

Bargaining

Among all the medical appointments and the organizing of files and records, parents eventually get faced with moments that allow for self-reflection and haunting self-doubt. The "what ifs" may consume us. We blame ourselves for not knowing what we could have done differently in order to prevent this from happening to our child.

Conversations with God are not uncommon in this stage. We would gladly commit to performing better in life for a good prognosis for our child. We wish this were happening to us instead of our child. We offer our higher power, or anyone else who will listen, that we would wear the back brace for our child and gladly undergo surgery if it meant sparing them this nightmare.

Depression

This is a natural and necessary step in the process of healing our grief. After all, it is a sad event in life for a child to be diagnosed with a condition that threatens their health, physical appearance, and psyche. This phase can feel like it will never end and there is a reducing prospect of hope.

Watching your child cry and not have a quick fix is quite difficult, but as parents we need to put our personal fears aside and model resilience. Talking about our feelings and getting our thoughts outside of our heads, which happens in the parents' support group at many Curvy Girls meetings, will provide the first steps toward healing.

Acceptance

This stage is not about accepting that everything is, or will be, "okay." Rather, it is about accepting the reality of our new, ongoing lifestyle with all its limitations, medical regimen, and challenges for our child and for us. The way we interact with our child, our spouse, other family members, and friends starts to hold a lot less intensity and general tension. Parents can talk a little more freely about their child's scoliosis. It is here that we can finally offer our child a respectable, more accomplished role model, one who can offer life examples of how setbacks and challenges are an unavoidable part of life. This, ironically, offers us opportunities to learn critical life skills. Acceptance can help you to segue into a new level of hope and human growth.

How we speak to our children helps them in the process of acceptance. Iyanla Vanzant discusses the power of Maya Angelou's words as, "Little energy pellets that shoot forth into the invisible realm of life. Although we cannot see the words, words become the energy that fills a room, home environment, and our minds." With this philosophy, the next time you take your child shopping for clothes, instead of saying you'll help her find clothes that HIDE her brace, suggest going shopping for clothes that will best COMPLEMENT her brace.

Simple changes in our words can have the biggest impact.

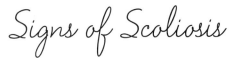

Signs of Scoliosis

Does your child have a hump when she bends forward? Does she have one shoulder higher than another? These are just a couple of the physical changes we commonly see, and may overlook. Below are signs to look for:

- Uneven hips or shoulders

- Waist asymmetry—one side of the waist may be straight and the other more curved

- Uneven creasing of lower back skin

- Leg length discrepancy

- Back pain

- Difficulty standing for long periods

- Trouble walking for long periods

- Leaning to one side

- Head off-center from trunk

- Protruding shoulder blade

- Noticeable hump on one side, flat on other side when bending forward

- Uneven breast development in girls

- Uneven skirt/dress lengths due to the unevenness in the hips

- Tendency to wear sweatshirts or oversized clothing

Preparing for Your Child's Medical Visit

THINGS TO CONSIDER WHEN CHOOSING AN ORTHOPEDIST:

- Is the orthopedist board certified in orthopedics?

- Do they specialize in scoliosis?

- How many children with scoliosis do they treat each year?

- How many adults with scoliosis do they treat each year?

- Do they belong to the Scoliosis Research Society?

- Do you know anyone whose child was treated by this physician? If so, how was their care and the doctor's "bedside manner?"

- Do they relate well to kids?

- Do they provide the ScoliScore® (saliva test)?

- Do they support conservative exercise treatment (Schroth Method or SEAS exercise)?

Parents and children can prepare together for medical visits. Make sure to ask your child what questions they may have. Children may need to be encouraged to ask their questions.

QUESTIONS TO ASK AT THE MEDICAL VISIT(S):

- How many curves?

- What are the curve degrees?

- What are the curve rotations?

- If the saliva test is provided, how are the results of the ScoliScore® used?

- What is the Risser score?

- How do you determine when my child is done growing?

- How often do you recommend x-rays?

- Do you use an alternative to x-rays, such as the DIERS Formetric 4D surface topography scanner for monitoring progression of scoliosis?

- If your child has pain, ask: *What might be causing the pain?*

- Can you recommend an exercise treatment program, such as Schroth Method or SEAS exercises?

- How often do you see your scoliosis patients?

- At what curve degree do you recommend surgery?

- Can you recommend a support group?

BRACING:

- How many hours a day do you brace your patients?

- Are all braces equal in terms of effectiveness for preventing curve progression?

- Is nighttime bracing an option?

- Are there physical side effects from bracing? Psychological side effects?

- Does bracing hurt? If it does, what should I do?

- How long is bracing?

- When do you begin brace weaning?

- If the brace is to be worn during school hours request a letter stating diagnosis and accommodations for removing and storing the brace, as well as anything else that will increase bracing compliance during school hours? *(See Advocating for Your Child)*

QUESTIONS TO CONSIDER AFTER THE VISIT:

- How did you feel about the visit with this orthopedist?

- Do you feel that all your questions and concerns were addressed, or did you feel rushed?

- Did you feel that your questions were answered in a way everyone understood?

- Did you feel confident in the care your child received?

- Was the office respectful?

- Was the orthopedist responsive to your concerns?

- Did the orthopedist relate to your child?

- How did your child experience the visit?

Bracing 101

A Conversation with Board Certified Orthotists Michael Mangino, CPO, CPed, LPO and Steve Mullins, CO

Michael Mangino founder and operator of Bay Orthopedics (www.bayorthopedic.com) is both a licensed and American Board Certified Orthotist and Prosthetist and a Board Certified Pedorthist. He holds several patents in the Orthotics and Sports Medicine field. His research has been published and he has been interviewed by various journals within the profession. He has served the profession as a founder and Board member of the New York Orthotics and Prosthetics Association and as an instructor to several of New York's universities.

Steve Mullins has been with M. H. Mandelbaum O&P since 1995 and received his ABC certification in 1998. Steve has taken many advanced courses in pediatric and spinal bracing. In 2000, he was one of the first practitioners certified in the SpineCor® dynamic scoliosis system in the U.S. and is certified in advanced software for evaluation and treatment.

Why bracing?

The purpose of bracing children with scoliosis is to stabilize the curve from progressing until the patient is finished growing in height. Bracing is not intended to reduce or correct scoliosis curves. The aim is to achieve a 50 percent reduction of curves while in the brace. This will be determined by an x-ray. There are cases where scoliosis curves have decreased even when out of the brace, but this is viewed as an exception and not the rule.

What is an orthotist?

An orthotist is a healthcare professional who provides care to patients with disabling conditions of the spine and limbs, by fitting and fabricating orthopedic devices (orthoses) under the direction and in consultation with physicians.

How to select a qualified orthotist?

Your orthopedist will provide you with the name(s) of orthotist(s). You may also want to check with other parents for their recommendations. It is important that an orthotist be board-certified in orthotics, and that they received additional post-graduate training in the use of scoliotic bracing. It is also beneficial for your orthotist to be trained in the use of several different types of scoliosis devices.

What should you expect from an orthotist?

The orthotist will examine and evaluate a patient's bracing needs in relation to their scoliosis. Often they will assist the orthopedist in the formulation of brace specifications. After fabricating the brace, the orthotist will evaluate the brace on the patient to assure fit, function, and quality of design. Your orthotist will determine a schedule to gradually implement bracing. However, it is your orthopedist who will determine the length and hours of bracing.

In addition to finding a qualified orthotist, it is important to ensure that the orthotist be able to establish a rapport with you and your child. Because brace compliance is a big issue with teen bracing, teens need to feel comfortable with their orthotist, and have trust in what they are saying. The orthotist needs to be able to hear and respond to your child's concerns in order to increase the likelihood of compliance. Your child will not wear their brace if it hurts. Orthotists should make themselves available to both parent and child for questions or problems related to bracing.

What can you expect from the new brace?

- A properly fitting scoliosis brace is snug.

- Bracing may be uncomfortable, but it should NOT hurt.

- There may be redness where the brace applies pressure. However, redness that does not clear in fifteen minutes after removing the brace, as well as sores or blisters, are immediate signs to contact your orthotist for a brace adjustment.

- Bracing should begin with a few hours a day, gradually increasing over several days until the recommended hours are reached.

Important: If pain is caused by the brace, return to the orthotist to determine the source of the discomfort. The pain should always be able to be relieved. **Irritation and pain caused by the brace is unacceptable.**

Bracing comfort tips:

- A shirt should be worn under the brace for both comfort and cleanliness. There are shirts made especially for this purpose, but they tend to be expensive. Most girls find that non-ribbed boys sleeveless undershirts work best.

- Witch hazel can be helpful to toughen the skin for brace contact.

- Talcum powder and a tee shirt should be used under your brace for added comfort.

What do all these words mean in relation to bracing: hard, TLSO, soft, custom-molded, casting, nighttime, bending?

There are a variety of braces available for treating scoliosis. Your orthopedist will determine which one is right based upon the type, location, and degree of the curves. Hard plastic braces used to treat scoliosis are considered *custom-molded.* In-brace reduction of the scoliotic curves can be achieved from the *casting* technique or from pad placement, depending on the style or orthosis prescribed by the physician. The orthotist replicates the affected area of a patient's body by a variety of means including making cast measurements, scanning the patient with laser scanners or photographic three-dimensional scanners, as well as orthometry methods.

Custom-made is custom fabricated. Molding or the computerized CAD/CAM program can accomplish this. Virtually every scoliosis brace is custom fabricated by molding the plastic over a corrected model of the patient.

Braces used to treat scoliosis include:
TLSO (Thoracolumbosacral Orthoses): a *TLSO* encompasses and supports the thoracic, lumbar, and the sacral spine.

- **Boston Brace:** the most commonly used TLSO brace; low-profile, made of lightweight *hard* plastic and padding, usually worn between sixteen- to twenty-three-hours a day. Strategically placed pads apply pressure to reduce and de-rotate the curves. The braces will have cut-outs and relief areas opposite the areas of the pressure pads to allow the braced curve reductions to occur.

- **Charleston Bending Brace®:** a *nighttime "bending brace"* made of molded plastic and padding, worn only while sleeping; designed to work in a shorter period of time by overcorrecting the primary curve by bending the curve in the opposite direction.

- **Providence Brace:** a low-profile plastic molded brace worn only while sleeping provides similar correction to daytime braces for mild to moderate curvature.

- **SpineCor® System:** a *soft*, tension-based TLSO made from cloth and elastic corrective straps used in low to moderate immature curves. Assists in retraining body posture for self-correction of the scoliosis curves. Must be worn for twenty hours a day.

- **Rigo System Cheneau Brace (RSC)®:** a three-dimensional brace, unlike most TLSOs, the RSC® brace is not full-contact. This means it does not touch the body everywhere when it is applied to the person. Pressure is put on the prominences in all planes, and with "rooms" or spaces built on the opposite sides of the prominences. The convex areas have pressures, which allow the patient to move in conjunction with breathing exercises. This brace reinforces the correction that people learn while doing the Schroth exercises.

- **CTLSO (Cervicothoracolumbosacral Orthosis):** a *hard* plastic brace encompassing the cervical, thoracic, and lumbar spine.

- **Milwaukee Brace:** a full-torso brace that extends from the pelvis up to the base of the skull.

How do you keep your brace clean?

- The **inside foam** can best be sanitized by using rubbing alcohol on a gauze pad or an equivalent product. Paper towels work, but they usually suck up a lot of alcohol. The foam pads don't usually clean back to white because the body oils get into the cells of the foam. Windex® or Formula 409® will cut the greasy body oils somewhat, but the foam won't turn white again. Using a white tee shirt is the best protection for keeping the inside of the brace white, but there is really no reason why other light colors can't be worn. Sometimes brand new color shirts will stain the foam.

- The outer plastic of the brace will clean effectively with most household spray cleaners.

- The straps will eventually get a little yellow with body oils from grabbing the strap. Sometimes they will oxidize with sunlight. They can be cleaned pretty effectively if you soak them in a 50 percent bleach solution for a half hour, and then rinse them off with fresh water. You can either let them air dry or set a hairdryer on cool. If you use a hairdryer on heat, you will either ruin the Velcro or the strapping, and sometimes both.

Key Points to Remember about Bracing:

- Be your child's advocate.

- Never dismiss the importance of bracing.

- Remember to have your child follow a gradual course of bracing over several days.

- Brace adjustments should relieve any pain.

- Irritations and back pain caused by the brace is unacceptable.

- **Never allow a healthcare professional to intimidate you!**

Three-Dimensional Bracing
A Conversation with Orthotist
Grant Wood, MS, CPO (UK), CO (US)

Grant Wood specializes in three-dimensional bracing. He has the unique qualification of having trained and mentored with Dr. Manuel Rigo and Dr. Jacque Chêneau since 1995. Through the years, he has collaborated with them on numerous research publications, studies and workshops on the Chêneau Brace with the advanced Rigo principles. Grant Wood's professional career as an orthotist and prosthetist spans work in England, Spain, and his current U.S. West Coast practice in San Mateo, CA (www.align-clinic.com).

The following answers reflect Grant Wood's personal experiences, perceptions, and beliefs about bracing. Since each curve and patient's circumstances are unique, it is important to also consult your medical doctor, physical therapist and orthotist with any scoliosis questions.

How did the concept of three-dimensional bracing develop?
The concept of three-dimensional treatment for scoliosis has been used in Europe since E.G. Abbott first reported this in the Journal of Medicine in 1912. In the 1950s, Drs. Stagnara and Cotrel along with other scoliosis professionals reported positive 3D correction of scoliosis using plaster casting techniques. In 1979, Dr. Jacque Chêneau of France, inspired by these professionals, fabricated the original Chêneau Brace.

In the 80s and 90s, Dr. Rigo and Dr. Chêneau worked together and improved the original shapes to incorporate the derotational breathing techniques of Schroth physical therapy. Together they provided a brace design that did not increase the flatback but actually helped produce a more normal side view profile.

In the 2000s, Dr. Rigo redefined the brace using biomechanical concepts and the 3D principles enunciated originally by Chêneau and the other masters. The Rigo Classification of scoliosis and brace design uses the patient's clinical presentation (i.e., body shape) and x-rays to determine the patient's individual curve pattern. This furthered the brace shapes, designs and quality that have now been used for decades.

Knowledge of the 3D nature of idiopathic scoliosis has increased significantly during the last twenty years, and many scoliosis professionals have improved their individual techniques and quality as a result of this.

What is a three-dimensional brace?
A three-dimensional brace refers to the shape. When looking down into the brace you will see there are large expansion areas. The brace is designed with pressure and expansion areas built into the brace to provide correction in all three planes of the body—coronal, sagittal and axial planes. Without these expansion areas/rooms, you cannot achieve optimal 3D correction, an important component as this specific brace reinforces the correction that people learn while doing the Schroth Method exercises.

How does three-dimensional bracing differ in design from the standard TLSO?
The standard TLSO brace is more or less a full-contact and symmetrical brace, while the three-dimensional brace is not. The Chêneau Rigo-modified brace views scoliosis as a three-dimensional deformity, addressing all three planes, not just one. I have seen many cases in which professionals have pushed the thoracic curve so much (sandwich effect) that it was disadvantageous to the two other planes. Therefore, the concepts I use might accept less Cobb correction while improving corrections in the other planes and other curves. The Cobb angle is not less important to me, however, I am not going to negatively affect other planes (i.e., increase the flatback and rotation) and provide a poor clinical presentation at the cost of improved Cobb angle correction.

What is the specialized Chêneau Rigo-modified brace you make?
Approved by Dr. Rigo, the Chêneau Rigo-modified brace I design is called the Wood Chêneau Rigo (WCR) Brace. It has been modified

with the evolutionary concepts from both Dr. Chêneau and Dr. Rigo. From the years spent with both these experts, I have been able to create a specialized measurement technique, as well as brace shapes that provide patients with an orthopedic product that has optimum brace fit.

Do you just work with the three-dimensional brace?

No. As an orthotist, I have been trained to fit and fabricate all manner of braces for various conditions. My Master's thesis and my specialization is with the Rigo-modified Chêneau TLSO for scoliosis. I treat patients who have been prescribed Boston, Providence, Charleston, and other types of TLSO braces. However, with Dr. Rigo as my mentor, I made Rigo-modified Chêneau braces in Spain for eight years. This is the brace-type that most of my patients have and it is my preferred brace for most curves. This is not to say, by any means, that other TLSOs, if well-fitted and well-constructed are not efficacious. The Chêneau Rigo-modified braces, including the Wood Chêneau Rigo, is my choice because it addresses the three-dimensional nature of the curve, rather than just correcting the Cobb angle.

What are the most common clinical scenarios that you see when parents first contact you?

Unfortunately, most parents that contact me are usually in a crisis with their child's scoliosis. Often they are told that the brace their child has been wearing has failed and the curve has progressed from 40° to 55°. I also receive many calls from parents whose child is skeletally immature and on the threshold of surgery with a 38° to 44° curve. And lastly, I do have parents contact me for their child's first brace when the child is skeletally immature with a curve of 25° to 35°.

Can this brace be made for other types of scoliosis, such as congenital or infantile scoliosis?

Yes. I have had success making this type of brace for both congenital and infantile scoliosis patients. The brace design differs according to each patient's clinical situation.

Can you describe a couple of challenging corrections you were able to achieve with this type of brace for a child?

There have been many great corrections the WCR Brace has been able to obtain. One correction was a Cobb degree of 30° that achieved an in-brace correction of 2°, with an out-of-brace correction of 8°.

Another correction involved a four-year-old-boy diagnosed with infantile scoliosis. His curve was 76° when his mother first contacted me following a failed brace treatment. I was able to obtain an out-of-brace correction of 45°, along with a significant improvement in the clinical appearance of the child's spine. Now six years old, the child is doing well and has been able to avoid surgery up until this time. He has a much improved quality of life and scoliosis. Please note that this result is not always expected and does not necessarily mean that he won't require surgery in the future.

What would you consider a good in-brace correction?

That depends on the individual clinical presentation. For example, if a patient is more skeletally mature and presents with larger curves, it would be unrealistic to expect a 50 percent in-brace correction. It could happen but no one can promise this.

In-brace Cobb angle correction should not be the sole determining factor of how successful a brace is or is not because it only measures one aspect of the scoliosis curve. Too much focus on the in-brace Cobb angle result can lead to applying forces in a way that might improve the Cobb angle correction but negatively affect the scoliosis as a whole. This problem has occurred with non-bracing traction techniques as well.

How do you evaluate effective bracing?

We must evaluate the scoliosis in all planes, as a three-dimensional deformity. By the completion of the growth phase, the patient should present with a reduced Cobb angle or have stopped progressing, show improvement in trunk, shoulder and pelvic alignments, as well as display an accompanying change in their overall clinical presentation.

How does the three-dimensional brace you design address high thoracic curves?

The WCR brace has been able to treat the more challenging high thoracic curves, however, it must be noted that these curves are extremely challenging and difficult. We can treat curves at the T5 level, as well as address curves higher by adding a D modifier. A "D modifier" is an anterior piece of plastic that comes around to the opposite side of the curve below the collarbone. Another option for higher curves is the shoulder strap, which provides a counter force to the opposite (or concave) side of the curve. The shoulder strap is sewn webbing with a Velcro® padded strap. We use this in cases that used to be treated with the Milwaukee Brace or a TLSO with a hemi-cervical ring (CTLSO).

Is physical therapy recommended in conjunction with this brace?

Yes. The Schroth-based method of therapy, taught by Dr. Manuel Rigo at the Barcelona Scoliosis Physiotherapy School highly recommends this treatment as an adjunct to the Chêneau Rigo-modified brace. Many people now claim to treat scoliosis with Schroth therapy. I tell my patients to please make sure they are seeing someone who was trained and certified by the BSPTS, as Dr. Rigo has incorporated breathing exercises and postural corrections into his curriculum that work hand-in-glove with these of type of braces. Schroth-certified PTs can modify any exercise for a different TLSO, but the exercises were created and have evolved with the Chêneau Rigo-modified brace.

Exactly how does your brace function well with Schroth Therapy?

These braces have expansion chambers and windows built into the brace, allowing for a dynamic correction of the scoliotic deformities with each rotational breath that the Schroth-trained patient takes. In addition, areas of light pressure felt in strategic contact points remind the patient to adjust posture into an elongated or derotated position.

Can this brace be helpful for an adult with scoliosis?

Some young adults and adults have benefited from pain relief with a well-made brace. In adults, the objective is not correction, but pain relief and unloading of axial forces to the spine.

If someone travels to California for your brace, how often do they need to return for adjustments or for a new brace?
Families usually travel back once a year, depending on growth in height and in-brace x-ray results. We maintain contact and review the patient's condition every three months. I also spend a significant amount of time with each patient in the fabrication and fitting phase, so that the brace they receive will be, in my opinion, functioning optimally until significant growth occurs.

How do you continue to evaluate brace results?
I evaluate the effectiveness of the brace with subsequent brace fittings, follow-up photos, and in-brace x-rays, with frequent collaboration from the patient's orthopedic surgeon and physical therapist. This multi-disciplinary team approach optimizes the treatment and results, while ensuring that the patient always receives a brace that is comparable in quality to one that they would get if they traveled to Spain to see Dr. Rigo himself.

What is the role that Dr. Rigo has in the braces you design today?
Dr. Rigo provides consultation in patient diagnoses, brace designs, results and follow-up, which allows me to continually improve my patient care and results.

How good is compliance with the WCR Brace?
Because I trained and practiced in Europe for so long, my outlook on compliance is perhaps a bit different than that of some U.S. practitioners. Any brace that is actually creating a postural correction will have an adjustment period. How the parent and practitioner treat the discomfort during this period makes all the difference in the world between a successful brace experience and noncompliance with treatment. In Spain, for example, parents and practitioners emphasize the positive long-term outcome from wearing the brace faithfully. The child is empowered to do something positive for their body—wear the brace! This child accepts the brace and peers don't generally think much about it because the brace wearer doesn't project embarrassment about having to wear the brace. That said, my Chêneau Rigo-type brace wearers are typically compliance role models for all brace wearers.

__What's important to look for in an orthotist who is making a three-dimensional Chêneau Rigo–type brace?__
First and foremost it should be their reputation followed by individual skills, knowledge and experience. Any orthotist, no matter how good or certified they may be, will need years of experience to learn how to make a proper brace. However, an orthotist who makes a Rigo Brace (three-dimensional) must have many years of experience; otherwise, it would be easy to obtain less than favorable results. A scoliosis brace is not just an orthopedic product, but a device that is custom made. It has to be highly specific to correct in 3D the trunk and spinal deformities, just as the old masters had done. Therefore, if the orthotist hasn't been personally handmaking, fabricating and fitting the Rigo Chêneau Brace for at least five-to-seven years, on a regular basis, then I would question their ability to problem solve many situations that will occur. And lastly, remember a good name of a brace doesn't necessarily make it a good brace.

Advocating for Your Child

As parents, we have the responsibility for acting on behalf of our children and often being their voice. A child with scoliosis needs our advocacy not only with the physical and psychological effects of this condition, but also in the educational arena.

United States Federal Law, Section 504 of the Americans with Disabilities Act (ADA), protects the rights of students with any medical condition that affects their quality of learning environment. Students with scoliosis are, therefore, entitled to school accommodations under this law.

If your child is wearing their brace during school, parents need to ensure that certain provisions are made according to the child's particular needs. A physician's note must clearly specify the particular requests. At a minimum your child needs to be provided with extra time when they need to change clothes, and a "safe" and private place to go when they need to remove and store their brace. A child in a brace needs to have the ability to attend to their bathroom needs without drawing any unwanted attention. Their privacy must be respected and they should not be expected to "expose" their brace in front of peers until they are ready. It's difficult enough to wear a brace, so having to take it on and off during school hours is usually one of the girls' biggest worries.

Here are some of the items that have been included in the 504 Plans for students with scoliosis:

- Leaving class five minutes early to change in pre-designated private area, such as the school nurse's bathroom, prior to physical education class. Leaving physical education class ten minutes early to change clothes and get to next class.

- Leaving class three minutes early in order to avoid being pushed; maneuvering in a back brace can be difficult. Rushing through halls or stairwells can be potentially harmful for a child wearing a back brace.

- Provide an extra set of books at home so your child doesn't have to carry heavy books to and from school.

- Locker assignment should not require bending.

- Provide a safe place to store brace when not being worn.

- Air conditioner or fan placed in an overheated classroom might be required to help a braced child tolerate the heat. Back braces do not allow air flow and a child can easily become overheated.

- A child in a brace may need to get up out of their seat to stretch if sitting for extended periods of time.

- Avoid bus drills. No jumping out of the bus with back braces on.

- For tornado drills, squatting instead of bending over at the hips.

- If a school bus stop is far from your home, arrangements can be made to have your child picked up in front of your home.

- An elevator pass, if stairs are a problem.

- Physical Education activity should be modified based on what the child is able to do.

Teachers need to be advised of your child's scoliosis and bracing during school hours. Contact the teachers and educate them regarding your child's circumstances. If your child experiences back pain from scoliosis, prolonged standing or sitting will only exacerbate discomfort. Explain how important it is for them to show compassion and understanding when a student needs to get up and stretch due to the restrictiveness of the brace.

This was learned when Rachel Mulvaney encountered a less than understanding teacher who would not allow her to go to the nurse's office to remove her brace when experiencing muscle spasms. This situation left her feeling embarrassed and ashamed. Embarrassing a child or simply speaking in a curt manner can show a lack of understanding toward their situation. This alone can be enough for them to refuse to wear their brace to school.

Communication is key. Our job as parents is to ensure that the necessary information regarding our child's condition is shared with the appropriate people in their life.

Subsequently, if you find that you are not getting the necessary support, we encourage you to reach out to other professionals in the district, including administrators or the chairperson who oversees your child's 504 Plan.

It's essential for our children to feel supported and to know that "we have their backs," especially while they are being faced with the challenges of scoliosis.

Radiology 101
A Conversation with Raul Fuentes
Licensed Radiology Technologist

What is the difference between digital and conventional film x-rays?
Digital allows the technician to use less radiation, because it provides greater latitude for an acceptable and clear exposure. Digital exposures allow the doctor to enhance the contrast and/or density of the image once the exposure is complete and visible on the computer monitor screen. Then when adjusted, the doctor takes measurements for the scoliosis examination.

Can you explain how kids are protected during x-rays?
Kids and adults are protected by lead shielding, use of filters, and low radiation exposure. It is important for patients to remain still during the radiograph so as to avoid having to re-do an x-ray.

One of parents' biggest concerns is about radiation exposure for our daughters. Can girls' breasts and ovaries be shielded from exposure?
Lead shielding is used in an attempt to protect ovaries and breasts to the best of our ability. Because ovaries lie differently in each female, placing the shields too close to the spine could block the image and result in additional x-rays.

What should parents ask about when getting x-rays?
"Is an x-ray necessary at this time?" "Does the tech use shields, filters on the x-ray, and the lowest possible amount of radiation for an acceptable exposure?"

X-RAY THE SMART WAY

A parent's guide to minimizing radiation exposure for children who require scoliosis monitoring:

- Ask the Physician to Measure the Deviations with a Scoliometer BEFORE Referring to X-ray

- Demand Lead or Metal Shields on Breast and Reproductive Organs

- Make Sure the Patient's Back is Toward the X-ray Beam

- Ask the Radiology Tech to Use a Filter (Sometimes Called a Wedge)

- Have Patient Stand at Least 6 Feet from Machine

- Ask the Radiology Department to Use Narrow Beam Machine

- Ask the Radiology Department to Use Fast Conventional or Rare-Earth Films (because you don't need highest resolution to calculate Cobb angles)

Remember: You are Your Child's BEST Advocate

Courtesy of Scoliosis Rehab, Inc. (www.scoliosisrehab.com)

Introducing the
DIERS Formetric 4D

A Conversation with Patrick Knott, PhD, PA-C

Dr. Patrick Knott is a tenured professor at Rosalind Franklin University of Medicine and Science in North Chicago, IL. He has practiced as a Physician Assistant for over 20 years in the field of orthopaedic surgery, where he specializes in spinal deformity. His research has focused on ways to reduce radiation exposure in the pediatric orthopaedic population. He has over 50 peer reviewed journal articles, abstracts and scientific posters, as well as book chapters and continuing education programs to his credit. He is the lead researcher of a new multi-center project evaluating the DIERS Formetric system. For more information, visit www.sstsg.org.

What is the Diers Formetric 4D scanner?

The DIERS Formetric 4D scanner is a device that utilizes surface topography to analyze the shape of a patient's spine. The scanner projects stripes of light onto the patient's back. Then using a digital camera, a model of the spine can be reproduced without the use of radiation.

Can you give us a brief history of the scanner?

Helmut Diers of Germany developed the Formetric scanner in 1996. It utilizes the general principles of surface topography that have been used by researchers since the 1980s, but incorporates a unique algorithm to relate the surface topography to the 3D shape of the spine. It has been used extensively throughout Europe, and was introduced in the U.S. in 2010.

What is the clinical objective of having such a machine?

The clinical objective is to be able to follow the spinal deformity over time to see whether it is progressing. This has traditionally been done by physical examination and a series of spinal x-rays. However, the physical exam is not always very accurate in picking up small changes, and the x-rays expose patients to radiation that can have lasting side effects. The Formetric allows the clinician to accurately watch the deformity over time without any side effects.

During what stage of care would an orthopedic surgeon order this type of scan?

An x-ray will always be taken at the first clinical visit so the radiographic Cobb angle can be measured at that time. If a Formetric scan is also done at that time, the topographical measurements can be correlated with the radiographic measurements. Then in follow-up visits, as long as none of the topographic measurements change, we know that the radiographic measurements are likely not changing either, and follow-up x-rays can be avoided. If the topographic measurements do change over time, then that tells the clinician that a follow-up x-ray is necessary.

How does the scanner compare to an x-ray in terms of accuracy?

Many researchers have evaluated the reproducibility and accuracy of the scanner. One such article published in The Open Orthopaedics Journal, 2012, *"Comparison of Radiographic and Surface Topography Measurements in Adolescents with Idiopathic Scoliosis,"* concluded that the Formetric 4D is comparable to radiograph in terms of its test and retest reproducibility and thus, can reliably be used in the surveillance of patients with scoliosis.

What clinical information can benefit a patient who has scoliosis?

The latest version of this machine (4D) takes not only a static picture of the patient, but also a movie of the patient walking on the treadmill for an evaluation of spinal motion. This gives clinicians a whole new way to evaluate both spinal shape and spinal function.

Can the Formetric scanner benefit someone who has been fused?

Functional analysis will become especially important for the patient who has a spinal fusion. The motion of the vertebrae adjacent to the fusion is at the highest risk for disc degeneration, and this machine may be able to help the clinician identify abnormal movement at those levels earlier in time. It also allows us to study how spinal fusion effects gait and balance.

What role does the Formetric scanner have for a patient who is also doing Schroth exercises?

Physical therapists are now using the Formetric scanner to evaluate the effectiveness of their treatment. The patient can be scanned in their usual posture, and then again in several other positions to see how each movement effects the overall position of the spine. Because there is no x-ray or harmful effects, the therapist can scan the patient an unlimited number of times during Schroth or other similar therapy programs.

Where can parents obtain a scanning for their child?

There is a large multi-center group in the U.S. beginning an evaluation of the DIERS Formetric 4D system, and their work is described at the following website: www.sstsg.org. As more clinicians begin using the Formetric, it should become widely available for use in scoliosis surveillance. In the mean time, they may contact Diers Medical Systems for more information on the nearest clinician.

Families that live outside the United States who are interested in obtaining a scanning for their child can look on the Germany DIERS website, www.diers.de, for the closest distributor.

Do insurance companies cover this test?

This varies from state to state. Not all insurance companies understand this technology yet, so some cover the cost of a scan while others do not.

Surgery Tips:
Lessons Learned from Parents

TIPS FOR THE HOSPITAL

Promote scar healing. Dr. James Barsi tells us using a product called Medihoney® at the conclusion of surgery promotes wound healing. Ask your surgeon if they are willing to apply this.

The day of surgery—you and your child will go to pre-op. In some hospitals this is the same area as post-op. Here your child will be given a hospital gown in exchange for her clothing. An important tip that we were given was to ask the attending nurse if your daughter can keep on her underwear. This can be especially important to your daughter if she is menstruating.

Treat everyone with respect. "That goes for everyone, from the person who comes and empties the trash in your room to the doctor who performs the surgery. If you do, you will be treated the same way," advises Curvy Mom Patty Borzner.

Be your child's advocate. Do not be afraid to speak up on your child's behalf. Insist that everyone who comes to visit is healthy and washes their hands when they arrive. The last thing you or your child need is to get a cold or cough on top of everything else you're dealing with.

Help manage your child's pain. A pain medicine pump (PCA) should be arranged with your surgeon in advance. This allows your child to control their medication in response to pain. Pain needs to be managed. Leah, for example, never had to experience pain beyond what she could tolerate. "That's what pain medications are for," said Beth Roach, pediatric intensive care nurse. "Allowing the patient to 'bear the pain' is actually counterproductive and can prolong healing time. In order to heal, patients need to breathe deeply and move frequently, neither of which they can do while in pain."

SURGERY IS "BEHIND" YOU NOW

Don't sit on a recliner or a soft chair—it'll be too hard to get up, says Curvy Mom Debbie, whose daughter, Danielle, got stuck in one for more than an hour. "We had to put a hard dining room chair next to the recliner," Debbie explained. "Little by little, we were able to get our daughter from the recliner onto the hard chair. Once onto the chair, Danielle was able to stand.

Don't bend over soon after surgery. Debbie says, "When Danielle had to pick something up from the floor, she learned to drop slowly to her knees, get what she wanted and then rise back up the same way."

Use slip-on shoes rather than ones with laces. Bending down is difficult, and that includes bending down to tie shoes.

Go slow getting up from bed—and ask for help if needed. Start by setting up the bed far enough away from the wall so that you can walk on both sides. That way, a parent or caregiver can lend a hand. Mom Debbie says, "I bent down so Danielle could hold onto my shoulders as I stood up. In this way, she was using my leverage to stand." Getting into bed can be tough, too. To ease the task, Danielle's parents built her a small but sturdy wooden platform that she could step up on. The platform allowed her to get further back onto the bed with less scooting and sliding.

Consider using hospital-type "chuck pads" for moving your daughter to the edge of the bed. The plastic on the bottom moves easily across the sheets, allowing you to pull your child towards you without much effort on her part, or yours.

Think about moving that bed to the first floor because it means less stair-climbing—and puts your "patient" closer to the action. Since Leah's room was upstairs, her parents opted to temporarily set up a hospital bed on the first floor. That meant Leah wouldn't have to worry about climbing stairs and that she would be closer to family members during the day.

A hospital bed can make things easier. While not necessary, the hospital bed's incline and side rails helped Leah to be more self-reliant when getting up. Her mom, Robin, slept on the couch next to her just in case anything was needed in the middle of the night. Insurance companies will pay for a hospital bed if your surgeon prescribes it.

Think outside the box when it comes time for a shower. Once your child is able to have her hair washed, you will not want her standing for very long. Robin's neighbor came up with the idea of using a light-weight aluminum lawn chair rather than a surgical seat for her daughter Leah's showers. The lawn chair proved less cumbersome than a medical shower chair. Remember, the incision can't get wet until all the bandages, known as Steri-Strips™, fall off. Robin used a large plastic garbage bag and put a hole in the bottom for Leah's hair and head to come out and be washed—like the Caped Crusader on a Lawn Chair!

Read and follow the instructions for all pain medications. Surgical patients will go home with a prescription for oral pain medication. Robin realized too late that she was giving Leah the same amount of medication that she was getting in the hospital—twice what the surgeon had prescribed. It was only when Leah started running out of pain medication that her mother read the instructions and realized her mistake.

PART V
STRAIGHT TALK

A Conversation with
Dr. John Labiak

Board certified orthopedist, **John Labiak, MD,** specializes in all aspects of pediatric and adult spinal surgery, including degenerative conditions, trauma, and tumors, with special expertise in complex pediatric and adult spinal deformity. Presently, Dr. Labiak is the Clinical Assistant Professor of Orthopedic Surgery and Neurosurgery at Stony Brook University Hospital.

Dr. Labiak is a member of the Scoliosis Research Society, the American Academy of Orthopaedic Surgeons and the Medical Society of the State of New York. He was listed as a Health Grades five-star medical doctor and by Castle Connolly Medical Ltd. as one of the top orthopedic surgeons in the United States.

HOW TO FIND A SPINE SPECIALIST

How do parents find a good orthopedic doctor who specializes in scoliosis?
Dr. Labiak: I think for scoliosis, in particular, the Scoliosis Research Society is something you'd want your doctor to belong to. The SRS is actually a very good society because it's exclusive, meaning that they just don't allow anyone to join. First, you have to qualify. You have to be board certified, in practice for a certain amount of years, actively practicing in spinal deformity, and prove that a percentage of your practice is in this specific field. You also have to present a couple of papers on research to qualify. You don't have to be a member to visit www.srs.org and use their physician locator.

Another way to find a doctor in this field is to obtain a recommendation from someone that you trust. I don't think an institution matters as much. I've seen great people at a great institution and horrible people at a great institution. And then, I've seen great people in not such a great institution, so the institution is less important than the person. The bottom line is that the best recommendation is always from another person who has intimate knowledge of that physician.

What led you to become an orthopedic surgeon, more specifically, in spine disorders?

Dr. Labiak: I'm an engineer by training. My undergraduate degree is in chemical engineering. So an unusual path led me to medicine. Scoliosis is very intriguing and challenging from an engineering standpoint. I think it was almost natural for me to get into scoliosis just from that.

Explain how engineering and scoliosis are linked together for you.

Dr. Labiak: Your spine is a flexible column and so everything that applies to a flexible column in a building or in some other structure applies to your spine as well. Having a biomechanics background is very beneficial because you can choose the implants more objectively and carefully, based on what they are able to do. Something as simple as choosing the metal used for the scoliosis surgery, such as titanium, cobalt chrome, or stainless steel, all ties in and helps the decisions I make because of my background.

Why do some kids who compliantly wear their brace still end up requiring surgery?

Dr. Labiak: That's the hundred-thousand-dollar question. Hopefully, the saliva test will help. The new genetic testing, the ScoliScore® test by Jim Ogilvie, indicates that there is some genetic marker that would show up in a certain subset of patients to indicate an increased risk of scoliosis. This test can only offer the likelihood of progression; it does not guarantee that there will be no curve progression.

DNA TESTING

ScoliScore® is a sample of saliva taken from a patient and compared to a large genetic database of scoliosis patients that Axial Biotec maintains. After analyzing the genetic markers contained in saliva, a score from 1-200 is generated. It is this score that helps to predict the risk of curve progression.

A ScoliScore® from 1-50 is considered low risk for curve progression, 51-180 moderate risk, and 181-200 more significant risk for progression.

Would bracing still be necessary if a child has a low Scoliscore®?
Dr. Labiak: Your question is, "Would you put someone in a brace that would have not progressed anyway, and at the end they end up no better than having not worn the brace?" I think bracing clearly has a positive effect on reducing the number of kids who progress to the point of needing surgery.

What if the ScoliScore® is higher?
Dr. Labiak: I think it's basically for informational purposes. I would still continue to treat that person the same way.

Is there always a genetic component in scoliosis?
Dr. Labiak: No, not always. If, however you do have a first-degree relative who has idiopathic scoliosis, your risk of having a curve increases by ten times, but not your risk of having an operative curve.

Does an eleven-year-old child with a 35° curve and a zero Risser have what is considered a "big curve"?
Dr. Labiak: If you have a new patient who is eleven, has a 35° curve without any development of secondary sex characteristics, whose tri-radiate cartilage is open, absolutely, that's a big curve.

What is your treatment protocol?
Dr. Labiak: Every single patient is an individual. A lot of people refer to it as an art rather than a science because it's so fluid. So you'll hear all the time that people who present with a curve greater than 25° and growth remaining are candidates for bracing. Also, people who have curves of 40° and who are still growing, or have progressed despite bracing, would be a candidate for surgery. It's even more complex than that. It really depends upon the whole child. What is their skeletal maturity? What is the magnitude of their curve? How has the curve behaved?

I've been able to take many children whose curves were 40° or more, had growth remaining, and not had to operate on them.

How are you able to accomplish that?
Dr. Labiak: As doctors, we have observation, bracing, and surgery. Most of those patients would stay in a brace until they finish growing. But my point is, if you have somebody who is still growing but

is at the end of their growth, and they have a 40° or 45 ° curve, that's still not the end of the world. You can still get that patient to skeletal maturity with a curve less than 50° and they may live happily ever after without surgery.

BRACING

Which brace do you usually recommend for your patients?
Dr. Labiak: My first recommendation would always be the Boston Brace. It's probably the most popular brace I recommend because it has the best and longest track record. If the child looks like they're going to give me a hard time, then I'll go to the SpineCor® or nighttime bracing, which is either the Providence or Charleston®.

Are the reports on the SpineCor® bracing good?
Dr. Labiak: The results that are published so far have been reasonably good and comparable.

Does the SpineCor® have guidelines on who can use it?
Dr. Labiak: Absolutely. You cannot be over a certain degree to be able to use this type of bracing. Despite the fact that you would think that kids would like it more, my experience has been that most kids like it less because of the pelvic attachment.

When do you recommend the nighttime brace?
Dr. Labiak: The curve has to be of a moderate degree and it also has to be flexible. The first thing I do with a nighttime brace is to have them get an x-ray in the brace. If they don't correct substantially, I won't use it, because their results are not going to be acceptable.

As far as nighttime bracing goes, I usually use that for my most resistant patients who are the least compliant. If I have a child who I am convinced will not wear a brace during the day, I would consider a nighttime brace for that patient.

What type of correction can you get from the nighttime braces?
Dr. Labiak: The Charleston® is a bending brace. The Providence is slightly different; it is really an overcorrection brace. The Charleston

Brace® actually bends the trunk in the opposite direction, where the Providence Brace overly corrects the curve.

Why can't the Boston Brace be used as a nighttime brace?

Dr. Labiak: If you only wear the Boston Brace at night, the effectiveness is not going to be what you want. Part of the intuitive way a nighttime brace works is by overcorrecting the curve. So you're taking this curve and really straightening it out. If you ask any of these kids to stand up while in this brace they would look a little off balanced.

Why wouldn't we want to have the kids wear two types of braces—one for daytime and one for nighttime?

Dr. Labiak: It's a valid question that doesn't have studies to prove or disprove.

When do you brace your patients?

Dr. Labiak: This is sort of a gray scale. It goes back to the art. If someone came in with a 25° curve with a zero Risser, most probably that child is going to be braced. Every child is an individual, so you try to make an accurate assessment of their growth potential. You look at how tall their parents are and their Risser stage (which measures your pelvis growth plate). You would look at their triradiate cartilage (which measures your hip growth plate) and your bone age (x-ray taken of your wrist). It is then compared to something called Greulich Pyles atlas where we can compare your bone age to your chronological age to determine whether you are lagging behind your peers as far as growth. The Risser sign is the most used for scoliosis but, unfortunately, it is a relatively poor indicator of growth.

Where is your Risser located?

Dr. Labiak: The Risser sign is in your iliac, your pelvis growth plate. By monitoring this growth plate, it helps determine how much growth remains in the spine.

Is there a difference between how you would monitor boys versus girls?

Dr. Labiak: If a girl has a moderate curve, and reaches a Risser 4, her risk of progression reduces dramatically. However, where boys are concerned, this is not necessarily true. When we're treating a boy (and progression of scoliosis is less common in boys), we look at the Risser sign a little differently. When a girl grows, she'll grow dramatically and then stop. The boys will have a dramatic growth spurt and will then continue to trickle along for a couple of years.

Practically speaking, we have studied both boys and girls, and boys' curves can continue to progress at a Risser 4. Therefore, boys need to reach a Risser 5 before we tell them to stop bracing.

How and when do you determine that your patient is ready to be weaned?
Dr. Labiak: Before I make this decision, I would take these signs into consideration: the Risser sign and the triradiate cartilage. You can have Risser of zero, but if your triradiate cartilage is closed, you might be further along in your growth.

How many hours do you recommend that your patients wear a Boston-type brace?
Dr. Labiak: The Boston-type brace shows very little difference in effectiveness from sixteen hours or twenty-two to twenty-three hours a day.

What is this information based upon?
Dr. Labiak: There have been studies that have shown that there is no real difference in effectiveness between sixteen hours versus twenty-two hours per day bracing. And the truth is, we're treating people, young people, and if the brace ends up in the corner it's not doing anyone any good. I think you really need to assess the child and the parents and their relationship. There are kids that will wear a brace for twenty-three hours a day and not blink an eye. They'll do it and there's never a real issue. And then there are kids who absolutely, positively will not do it. They'll use it as a wedge between them and their parents, which is not anything negative against the child. It's just a difficult time in their life. But I think you have to make an assessment of that to some degree. I'd rather have a kid wear a Boston-type back brace for sixteen hours a day and wear it, than have a kid who is told to wear it twenty-three hours a day and hides it in their locker. Again, for me, the difference in effectiveness is not worth the difference in compliance.

What is your approach to getting your patients to comply?
Dr. Labiak: It is difficult. The best thing I could do is try to establish a relationship with the child, not be their best friend, but try to convince them that the brace is for them, not for their parents, and not for me. If you could convince them the brace is for them, they can exert control over their condition and then I find they usually wear it. I would also try to establish a relationship with the parents, too, so that we have a strong, three-way partnership. I think wearing the brace for sixteen hours a day is a huge shift from twenty-three hours a day with those difficult kids.

Can someone's curve decrease after they are braced?
Dr. Labiak: It's rare, but it can happen. A brace is really meant to stop progression; it's not meant to correct or reverse the curvature. Having said that, everybody who treats scoliosis can tell you about two or more patients who were treated with a brace, started out with x curve and ended up an x minus 20° curve, and we don't really know why. However, in the majority of cases, bracing is to hold the progression of the curve.

How long do you want your patients out of brace for follow-up x-rays?
Dr. Labiak: Twenty-four hours.

Is a girl who is two years post-menarche with a Risser 4-5 done growing?
Dr. Labiak: Yes, you're done with your longitudinal growing.

Can curves continue to progress after skeletal maturity?
Dr. Labiak: There have been really two major studies. The Italian study and the Iowa long-term study both looked at progression of scoliosis in untreated patients who were skeletally mature. They broke it down into different curve types, thoracic versus lumbar. The results indicated that most curves over 50° progressed, while curves under 30° did not. This gave us some of the guidelines. For instance, if a child is 30° or less when they are skeletally mature, their prognosis is excellent; they're essentially out of the woods. The people who are above 50°, I would keep an eye on them.

So you don't necessarily operate on someone who has a 50° curve?
Dr. Labiak: If they are skeletally mature, I might. Again, it varies from individual to individual. I also might let that individual prove to me they are going to progress. And if they did progress, I would recommend surgery for them. A part of my reason is that a small percentage of those people will not progress, and you won't have to do an operation on them. The other thing is if you operate on someone at 50° versus 55°, there is no difference in the ultimate outcome. But at 50° and above, I will tell a patient that there is a significant risk to progress.

Is that because of the effect of gravity?
Dr. Labiak: We don't understand it completely, but from an engineering standpoint if you have a column and it's deformed and curved, when it reaches a certain magnitude it wants to collapse; that collapse is really the effect of gravity, like a stack of dominos.

It sounds like you are conservative in your approach to surgery.
Dr. Labiak: I plant the seed about surgery just so people think about it as a possibility. In my mind what I'm trying to prevent is a poorer ultimate outcome based on waiting too long. I don't worry about a child going from 40° to 45° versus 50° to 55° because if that happens under my watch it has not changed their ultimate outcome. I can still have that child with the exact same outcome at the end.

Do curves progress from pregnancy?
Dr. Labiak: No. Years ago there was a study that showed no significant progression during pregnancy. People thought the hormones that allow your pelvis to open up to deliver a six-, seven- or eight-pound child would also allow the ligaments in your spine to become lax enough to let the scoliosis progress. There was only one study that seemed to show progression, but other studies have since refuted that. I tell my patients when they're pregnant not to worry about progression and they can even have an epidural without difficulty.

Can a fused patient have an epidural?
Dr. Labiak: It depends on where they're fused to, however, most patients can.

PAIN

We have some children in our support group who suffer with physical pain from their scoliosis. They cannot stand for long periods or walk long distances. When their complaints are brought to their doctors they are told there is no pain associated with scoliosis. How can this be?

Dr. Labiak: For those kids who are in pain, they will usually get better. So you're not talking about a chronic situation. Ultimately, when you look at them when they're fifty or sixty years old and compare them to their peers they're going to be exactly the same. So it's a short-term phenomenon. Typically, the pain doesn't last.

Do you think doctors should ask if their patients have pain?

Dr. Labiak: Yes. I will always ask my patients if they have pain. Do they have pain every day? Do they take anything for their pain? Do you take Advil® or Tylenol®? Does it help? All of these questions will help me understand what pain they're experiencing.

Is the pain due to the imbalance in their body?

Dr. Labiak: It's probably multi-factorial. Some of the girls that are braced have some atrophy and their core is not as strong as it should be or could be. I think the real reason you hear there is no pain, is because if somebody has pain with scoliosis, it warrants making sure that it's not something else. That doesn't mean you can't have pain, but if you have pain you should make sure it's not something more serious, like a tumor or syrinx.

The most common structural reason to have back pain as an adolescent is spondylolysis, a fatigue fracture between the superior articular facet and inferior articular facet.

This condition doesn't have anything to do with scoliosis then?

Dr. Labiak: There is a slightly higher risk of this problem with scoliosis patients. When we do MRIs or bone scans we are looking for spondylolysis or a benign tumor that can cause scoliosis. So when we have a patient who has pain, you want to make sure it's reproducible pain. You want to make sure that the patient doesn't have anything else going on like a syrinx—a collection of cerebral spinal fluid within the spinal cord. This is actually a common reason for someone to be misdiagnosed as having idiopathic scoliosis, when in fact they have some underlying condition.

Which test has the highest radiation?

Dr. Labiak: A CAT scan has a tremendous amount of radiation. So I will do my best not to put a skeletally immature adolescent through this because of the extremely high dose of radiation they would be exposed to.

For what reason would you order an MRI for your patient?

Dr. Labiak: There would be several reasons. For one, if you have a curve that is not playing by the rules, meaning you have a curve that is convex to the left in the thoracic spine instead of following the majority of curves, which are convex to the right. Not only does a little light bulb go off but those kids need to be imaged. If you have a patient who has night pain or night sweats, or reproducible pain, these symptoms warrant that a patient be imaged. Recently, papers at the Scoliosis Research Society suggested kids with bigger, stiffer curves have an MRI to rule out underlying conditions causing the scoliosis, for instance a syrinx. You certainly would want to know about it because it changes the way you would correct the curve and sometimes it might warrant treatment of the syrinx.

Years ago, I had a very interesting case with a young girl from Ukraine who had lived relatively close to Chernobyl. Her family was very sensitive to the idea of radiation so they didn't want her to have too many x-rays. She had scoliosis with back pain and night pain. This is not typical back pain; it woke her up out of sleep at night. While treating her scoliosis, I then suggested we order a bone scan because I wanted to make sure she didn't have anything else going on. Her family refused explaining they were afraid she was already exposed to too much radiation. Ultimately, after a while I gained their trust and I was able to convince them to let her have the bone scan. Sure enough the bone scan lights up like a Christmas tree; she had a benign tumor—osteoid osteoma. She also had a big curve, around 35° to 40°. There are many ways to treat osteoid osteoma today. We did microsurgery back then, removed the tumor, and afterwards her scoliosis improved completely.

So how does that make sense from an engineering standpoint?
Dr. Labiak: The reason why people get scoliosis from an osteoid osteoma is totally different than an idiopathic scoliosis. Basically, in her case it was a mechanical issue. She had muscular spasms, which started the curve progression. Once you get rid of the stimulus and allow the muscles to relax, a normal state can return to her spine. The reason I shared this story is that it highlights the fact that you want to make sure where the pain is coming from.

PHYSICAL THERAPY

Do you suggest physical therapy while braced?
Dr. Labiak: I do discuss some kind of therapy with all my patients, because ultimately I think they should stay active. I won't force the issue because I believe in the end it all balances out. If you have a child in a brace for a couple of years, their core muscles will certainly become atrophied a little bit, but once they get out of the brace they make that up relatively quickly.

Can the child regain core muscle strength after spinal fusion?
Dr. Labiak: Absolutely, but more slowly than a braced patient.

SURGERY

Do you take cosmetics into consideration when you make your decision regarding surgery?
Dr. Labiak: Absolutely. When I refer to the ultimate outcome, cosmetics are a part of it. When I treat a patient with scoliosis, I am concerned about their cosmetics, and it's a big concern of theirs as well. Frankly, many curves are cosmetically fine, especially balanced curves. I think your eye actually likes curves. However, if you have someone with a highly rotated curve or who is decompensated, that might be cosmetically less pleasing. I would take that into consideration.

If I cannot achieve the same results, the same ultimate outcomes, then I start to think about treating that person earlier, rather than later. I want to get the best cosmetic, functional outcome.

How do you decide which metal you would use?
Dr. Labiak: A lot of that depends upon the patient that you are dealing with, the curve, its magnitude, and its flexibility. So if you have a really stiff, large curve, you want to use a metal that is more rigid and stiffer, like cobalt chrome or stainless steel because that will help you correct the curve better. If you use something like titanium, which is a little bit more flexible, you're not going to get the same correction because of the nature of the material.

There are also tradeoffs because titanium has better imaging characteristics than either cobalt chrome or stainless steel. If you have a smaller curve, or are less rigid, you might want to use titanium because you could image those patients better, particularly in an MRI down the line.

Does having metal in your back prevent you from having an MRI?
Dr. Labiak: No, not all. Really what they're talking about with MRIs is ferromagnetic metals. These are metals that would stick to a magnet, so you can have an MRI without difficulty with any non-ferromagnetic metal in place. The only issues are that it does distort the MRI images locally. But let's say you had a T5 to T12 fusion, and you need an MRI of your brain or your knee, you can absolutely have this done safely. There's a lot of confusion about this. I receive calls about this all the time from patients who have had spine surgery and now have to have an MRI. "Can I have this safely?" And the answer is universally, yes.

How often does a patient's fusion fail?
Dr. Labiak: The rate for adolescence fusion surgery success is actually pretty high, in the 90th percentile bracket.

Are there any side effects with corrective surgery?
Dr. Labiak: Kids fused in the lower lumbar spine (L4, L5) have more of a tendency to back pain as adults, than kids that are fused higher. We try to fuse as few segments as we can, especially in the lower spine. The upper (thoracic) spine doesn't really matter as much because it is usually rigid to start with, so there's not a lot of force transmission that occurs compared to the lower (lumbar) spine.

How long do you follow patients post-surgery?
Dr. Labiak: I will follow them for a couple of years.

STAPLING

Can you explain the surgical process of stapling?
Dr. Labiak: What they are trying to do is to suspend or inhibit the growth on one side of the curve, while allowing growth to continue on the other side of the curve.

What type of scoliosis patient would be a candidate for this procedure?
Dr. Labiak: In order to be a candidate for this procedure, you have to have a moderate curve. You cannot have a big curve; it's not as effective and you need growth potential remaining.

Is it true that there are only a small percentage of children who can have this procedure?
Dr. Labiak: Yes, that is correct. This is why it's important that you stick to the fine guidelines on who is a candidate, especially since it's a relatively new procedure. This procedure is not going to be the treatment for every curve.

Do the staples ever come out?
Dr. Labiak: No, it's permanent.

Does stapling eliminate bracing?
Dr. Labiak: That is correct; there is no bracing.

SCHOOL SCREENING

What do you recommend be done at school screenings?
Dr. Labiak: I've actually talked to many school nurses over the years and I strongly recommend the use of a very simple tool, the Scoliometer. They ask the child to bend forward and you put this over the spinous process and it basically tells you how many degrees ATR (angle of trunk rotation). William Bunnel has a couple of studies using this simple device and determined that if your angle of trunk rotation is less than 7°, there's a 98 percent likelihood that your curve would be less than 20°.

Why isn't this being used then?
Dr. Labiak: Good question. I have been encouraging them to do this.

Is this an expensive device?
Dr. Labiak: No, it's only about $40.00 and it's very easy to use.

How can someone pass a school screening test and still have scoliosis?
Dr. Labiak: A thoracic curve is more obvious than a lumbar curve because your thoracic spine is attached to your ribs, so when your thoracic spine rotates, your ribs pop up. Since your lumbar curve doesn't have ribs, it makes it more difficult to see the rotation of the spine. However, it would be seen when using this device.

My point is, if you're going to have a school screening, you might as well have an effective school screening. If you have an ineffective school screening, it does two bad things. First, it gives a child a false sense of security, and two, it over-refers people. So we take people who don't have scoliosis and send them to doctors. Parents take off from work, the child takes off from school, they bring their child to the doctor, get an x-ray, have x-ray exposure, pay for the expense of an x-ray, and find out there's nothing wrong.

A Conversation with
Dr. Laurence E. Mermelstein

Laurence Mermelstein, MD, is a Board Certified Orthopedic Surgeon whose clinical practice places an emphasis on pediatric scoliosis and deformities, adult degenerative deformities, and minimally invasive surgical techniques. As the first surgeon on Long Island to perform the Posterolateral Endoscopic Discectomy procedure, he continues to be on the forefront of surgical technology. He has lectured extensively at national and international meetings regarding Spinal Biomechanics and Instrumentation and has authored numerous papers and book chapters related to spinal issues. (www.lispine.com)

What led you to specialize in scoliosis?

Dr. Mermelstein: I was initially drawn to orthopedic surgery as a specialty. I enjoyed being able to definitively "fix" patients and make a large impact on their quality of life. The technology of the field attracted me as well. I enjoy seeing patients that span the gamut from child athletes to senior citizens. I was intrigued with spinal surgery as a sub-specialty, as it is probably the most challenging of the orthopedic subspecialties. The opportunity to make a huge difference in patients, who many times think they cannot be helped, is precious. The potential complications are quite high, and there are some days that I wish I was doing something else, but I guess everyone could say that at some point.

Why don't we know what causes adolescent idiopathic scoliosis?

Dr. Mermelstein: It is likely that a number of different genetic and environmental factors are involved in the development of scoliosis in any given patient. Adolescent idiopathic scoliosis appears to be highly dependent on genetics, as well as to the unique biomechanics of the human spine.

Have any of your patients taken the ScoliScore® saliva test? What is your opinion of this test?
Dr. Mermelstein: Yes, some of my patients have taken the test. Unfortunately, I find it hard to interpret. Kids are scoring in the middle, and at this time we don't know what that means. We await further studies on kids who have already been braced and who have also been fused. This will give doctors a better idea of how to interpret the score.

What do you do when a child complains of pain?
Dr. Mermelstein: There usually is no pain associated with idiopathic scoliosis, but if a child complains I will assess the problem to make sure nothing more serious is going on. If everything is fine, that child might benefit from some physical therapy.

Can heavy backpacks cause or worsen scoliosis?
Dr. Mermelstein: There is no scientific evidence that scoliosis is caused by backpacks. A heavy backpack may contradict the effect of a brace on scoliosis, and in these cases should be limited.

Is it possible that although it's called "adolescent" scoliosis that it may have existed undetected years before? Is it just the adolescent growth spurt that makes scoliosis more apparent?
Dr. Mermelstein: By definition, idiopathic scoliosis is not present at birth. Again by definition, it is first detected in kids, ten- to sixteen-years of age. If the curve is seen before ten years of age, it is termed "juvenile" or "early onset" idiopathic scoliosis. The earlier that the curve presents, the more likely the curve will progress. It is with the rapid growth acceleration that occurs with puberty that the magnitudes of these curves sometimes increase rapidly.

Other than the classic rib "hump" upon bending, what are some of the other earlier common signs of idiopathic scoliosis that parents can be aware of?
Dr. Mermelstein: One can see shoulder asymmetry, elevation, etc. Look for scapula asymmetry, waist asymmetry, chest, or sternal asymmetry. Forward bending highlights the ROTATIONAL component of scoliosis in the thoracic (ribs) and lumbar (flanks).

BRACING

Why is there a discrepancy among orthopedic spine surgeons regarding the number of hours for brace wear (sixteen hours versus twenty-three hours)?

Dr. Mermelstein: Research has shown that the more time in the brace, the better. The efficacy is "dose" (time) dependent. To my knowledge, there is no "threshold" time above which it is not helpful or even counter-productive. My experience is that, in kids, we shoot for twenty-three hours a day, realizing the actual time will be much less, accounting for bathing, swimming, sports, and gym class.

Full-time bracing in your practice is twenty-three hours. Are there exceptions?

Dr. Mermelstein: As far as the amount of hours they need to brace, I try very hard not to give them a number. I will tell them full-time bracing means they wear it all the time except for when they shower, exercise, or do any other activity such as sports or dance. The bottom line is, the more they wear it, the better the results. I always remind them the best time to wear it is when they're not doing anything.

Are there any exceptions? Yes. Depending on the child, and their curve, I might suggest nighttime bracing. The Charleston Bending Brace® has very good results. The compliance is also very good and all they need to do is sleep in it for eight hours a night.

If a child had a 20° curve, would you begin bracing as an early intervention?

Dr. Mermelstein: Not usually, I probably would just continue to monitor that child. I don't like to put a child in a brace any earlier than I have to. If the patient is seventeen years old and four years post-menarche, there are no reasons to brace. However, if there is evidence of family history of scoliosis, I might be more aggressive. If I have an eight-year-old child who has a rather stiff curve, and whose mother and grandmother had surgery on their scoliosis, I would intervene with bracing sooner.

When do you decide your patient needs to go to full-time bracing?
Dr. Mermelstein: I usually will start full-time bracing when the curve reaches 25° and the child still has a lot of growth remaining. If for some reason I'm not sure about the growth remaining, I will send them for a bone age x-ray. The benefit of the wrist film is that it gives you a different angle on their bone age.

Literature has indicated that bracing over 40° is not effective. But in some cases we've observed, including Leah's, bracing continued even when she reached 47°. Can you explain?
Dr. Mermelstein: It is true that bracing is not as effective with curves over 40°, but this refers solely to the average patient. The reasoning is that curves over 40° usually continue to progress no matter what you do, thereby indicating the need for surgery. In addition, curves over 40° are usually quite stiff, and therefore resistant to bracing.

In some cases, I would continue to brace, especially in the very young patient who you want to grow more before fusion surgery. Or in the case when the patient is considering surgery, but not ready mentally or physically, I will brace to keep the curve as small as possible.

I had one case where we decided in February to do surgery in the summer and the child tossed the brace out. By the time we got to surgery, the curve progressed another 15°.

Parents worry all the time about kids losing their muscle strength because of wearing a brace all day. What do you recommend?
Dr. Mermelstein: For "full-time" braces, I recommend daily exercise outside of the brace for at least one hour. This could include gym class, after-school sports, dance classes, martial arts, and the like. Even if the child is not athletically inclined, I recommend that they find some physical activity to do. If the patient is very stiff, or has a neuromuscular impairment, formal physical therapy is recommended.

WEANING STAGE

What does the Risser 4 versus the Risser 5 indicate to the doctor?
Dr. Mermelstein: When a child reaches the Risser 4 it tells us that the growth in the spine has stopped, therefore, any additional growth that

can occur will come from their legs. When the child reaches Risser 5 the growth is complete; they've reached their final growth in height.

How long does it take for a child to go from a Risser 4 to a Risser 5?
Dr. Mermelstein: This varies. The range of completion is large: seven months to three-and-a-half years to reach a Risser 5. The average, however, is about two years.

Can curves continue to progress post-bracing? If yes, under what circumstances?
Dr. Mermelstein: Yes. Curves can progress after a brace is worn and growth ceases. I wish I could tell you why this happens in some patients and not in others. Many times, it has to do with the degree the curve winds up in after growth ends. Curves that are close to 40° and above have a higher likelihood of progression into adulthood, than curves less than 30°. That is why surgery is recommended for these larger curves; they do tend to progress, albeit at a slower rate than during puberty.

In addition, kids who are very compliant with bracing an aggressive curve may "just be delaying the inevitable," but that is impossible to tell when the bracing regimen begins.

SURGERY

Why does there seem to be discrepancy among surgeons as to what degree to surgically correct scoliosis? Can you describe typical scenarios requiring different recommendations?
Dr. Mermelstein: There is no absolute consensus regarding surgical indications for scoliosis. Indications for surgery are not based on degrees alone, although there is a general number of about 45°, give or take. The goals for surgery are correction, obviously, but equally important is to arrest progression. Not all 40° to 45° curves have the same risk. Thoracic curves are more likely to progress and the younger the patient the more likely surgery is suggested. A curve that is imbalanced is more likely to require surgery. Indications for adult scoliosis surgery are completely different, and more likely to require surgery for pain at a lesser degree. Different surgeons will be more or less surgically

aggressive and they each have their own reasons. It is the same for ALL types of orthopedic surgeries, arthroscopy to joint replacements.

Stapling is a newer procedure that is being done on younger patients who have taken the ScoliScore® and received a high score. What is your opinion on this procedure?
Dr. Mermelstein: If the only thing my patient has going against them is the result of a saliva test, then I'm not going to rush in and be aggressive. Stapling is an invasive procedure that does not have a long track record and does not guarantee correction of the curve. What happens when they get older and develop osteoporosis and the staples fall out? At least with fusion surgery, we have a hundred or so years of experience of what happens after a fusion surgery. With the staple procedure we have no idea how to handle a problem forty years from now. For me, there are too many "what ifs."

Can you explain the surgical procedure for stapling?
Dr. Mermelstein: This is a procedure performed through the chest where a large staple is placed across the convex side of the discs in the curvature. This retards the growth on the "short side" of the curve allowing the concave side of the discs to catch up. By definition, this surgery is for younger patients with smaller curves who have significant growth remaining in their spine. In other words, it is for patients who otherwise would be braced. The advantage is that they don't need to wear a brace. The disadvantage is that it is not a minor surgery (the thoracic cavity is entered). No long-term data yet; it is considered experimental.

How often do fusions not take/fail? Why can this happen?
Dr. Mermelstein: A failed fusion is called a **pseudoarthrosis** (literal translation—a "false joint"). Any fusion operation can result in a pseudoarthrosis. This can happen in a fusion operation as a consequence of too much motion at the fusion site (spinal hardware loosening) or a failure of biology; the bone failed to grow across the vertebrae. The attention to surgical technique can also minimize the pseudoarthrosis rate. Different types of bone grafts can influence healing rate (e.g., iliac crest bone graft is better than allograft —donor). A major

influence on healing rate is the condition of the patient. Medically speaking, the younger the patient, the smaller the pseudoarthrosis rate. Patients with diabetes and those on steroids are at higher risk. Smoking (nicotine) has a very detrimental effect on bone healing. Many times, pseudoarthrosis in kids' scoliosis surgery is asymptomatic and nothing need be done. Symptoms of a "pseudo" can be pain, loss of correction, or hardware failure and breakage. These symptoms may necessitate another surgery to repair the pseudo.

Anything the patient can do to prevent this?
Dr. Mermelstein: Patients need to heed their surgeon's instructions regarding activity levels post-operatively to not put excessive stress on the instrumentation. They should not smoke, and should have plenty of calcium and Vitamin D supplements, as necessary, if their diets are deficient. External bone growth stimulators, as prescribed by the doctor, can assist in high-risk patients.

Can you explain expansion rod surgery and when it might be used?
Dr. Mermelstein: Expansion rod surgery is generally used as a temporary procedure to hold aggressive curves in check in very small patients who have a lot of growth remaining. These patients either can't wear a brace, or the brace is not working, and are deemed too small to have a fusion surgery, which would stunt the growth of their trunk permanently. Usually, multiple surgeries are needed with this program and the complication rate is quite high. Repeated surgeries are needed over a course of years to elongate the rods as the child grows. Rod dislodgement rate, breakage, and infection rates are high. Eventually, the patient is converted to a traditional fusion surgery as a permanent correction.

What is an anterior fusion? Can you explain when this would be appropriate and what is entailed?
Dr. Mermelstein: Fusion surgery for scoliosis performed from the side is called an "anterior fusion." It is most frequently used for primarily lumbar curves. In this surgery, the entire disc is removed and the anterior ligaments released. This may allow for a better correction. Bone graft is put directly in between the vertebrae in the disc spaces.

Usually anterior instrumentation is put on the side of the vertebrae holding the correction until fusion is achieved. The advantage of this is that fewer vertebrae can be fused, especially lower down in the spine. Also, a selective lumbar fusion can be done, which is much less surgery. Lumbar and thoracic curves cannot be addressed with this approach at the same time. A separate surgical incision would be needed to address a thoracic curve at the same time; therefore, it is not usually done in double major curves (unless the curves are so stiff that they need an "anterior release").

Disadvantages are that the instrumentation fixation may not be as good anteriorly, as it is with pedicle screws posteriorly.

When making a decision about surgery for a child, what should parents look for in a hospital?
Dr. Mermelstein: The hospital has to be used to handling complex spinal procedures in the operating room with respect to anesthesia, instrumentation, and equipment. Cell Saver® blood scavenging needs to be available. Spinal cord intra-operative monitoring (IOM) needs to be available with staff experienced in these cases. The hospital needs to have a post-operative monitored care environment (ICU or "step-down") that is comfortable taking care of spinal surgery patients.

It is always helpful to be close to home so that post-operative complications can be handled in a timely fashion. It is nice that the parents can stay with the child as much as they desire (although I do recommend they get some quality sleep at some point!).

What are some things that you might recommend a child do prior to surgery to help get the best result?
Dr. Mermelstein: There are many things to do to prepare. Individually, each patient should be in as good physical shape as possible. Maximizing cardiovascular endurance will help in recovery and help minimize pulmonary complications. Skin hygiene is important (an issue in many adolescents). If acne is an issue in the surgical area, this needs to be addressed. Making sure the house is configured for easier recovery is important (make sure everything is on one level, if possible).

When doing a spinal fusion surgery, how do you select the rods that would be used for a particular patient?

Dr. Mermelstein: I have to take into consideration the type of curve it is. Is it a flexible curve or is it a large stiff curve? Since there are three different grades of titanium rods, I do try to use them whenever it's possible. The reason I consider this rod more often, is in case they need an MRI one day. The titanium rods will give better imaging results than stainless steel or cobalt chrome rods.

What is an intra-operative monitoring system during spine surgery?

Dr. Mermelstein: Intra-operative spinal cord monitoring (IOM) has become the gold standard for monitoring the function of the spinal cord during scoliosis correction surgery. Over the last ten years, the motor and sensory function of the spinal cord can be continuously monitored in real time during the surgery. Electrodes are placed on the patient's skull and in various muscles in the abdomen and legs. Impulses are sent to the brain and recorded in the muscles and vice-versa. Any intra-operative maneuvers or corrections that may impair spinal cord function can be reversed in a timely fashion, thereby minimizing post-operative deficits. Prior to the advent of IOM, a "wake-up test" was performed after the correction maneuvers and before the wound was closed. The patient was woken up while still on their stomachs during the surgery. If they had trouble moving their feet and legs, a spinal cord injury may be detected.

RECOVERY

While in the hospital, how will a parent be able to assess if their child's pain is being managed effectively?

Dr. Mermelstein: The patient should be able to roll from side to side and be able to get out of bed without a severe amount of pain. Pain cannot be completely eliminated, nor should this be the goal. If a patient is over-medicated, they will be overly sedated, and unable to participate in physical therapy and walking.

How soon after a child's spinal surgery do you recommend getting out of bed?
Dr. Mermelstein: The next day.

What do you recommend for scar reduction, when should it be started, and for how long?
Dr. Mermelstein: I have recommended a product called Scarguard MD®. It has a combination of silicone and vitamins and stays on for twelve hours before you pull it off and replace. This product is used once the new skin appears over the wound. It is not to be used on skin openings.

Within what period of time do you recommend patients be seen for the post-surgery office visit?
Dr. Mermelstein: I have patients return within two weeks of surgery mainly for a wound check, to make sure their wound is healing without infection. In addition, I get a standing PA (posteroanterior) and lateral x-rays full-length to check for overall balance, correction, and instrumentation placement. Most hospitals don't have the ability to take full-length x-rays.

Is it true that once a person has instrumentation in their spine that they should always be pre-medicated with an antibiotic prior to any dental visit?
Dr. Mermelstein: The ADA (American Dental Association) and the AAOS (American Academy of Orthopedic Surgeons) have put out a joint statement that routine prophylaxis for dental procedures is NOT necessary. Most surgeons will recommend delaying routine dental work for a period of time after surgery. There are higher risk cases (immuno-compromised individuals, patients on immunosuppressive agents), and higher risk dental procedures, where consideration may be given for antibiotics. But for the vast majority of patients, no prophylaxis is required.

DOCTOR-PATIENT RELATIONSHIP

What should a parent look for in an orthopedic surgeon when their child has scoliosis?

Dr. Mermelstein: I would recommend that they look for an orthopedic spine surgeon who has experience with both pediatric and adult scoliosis. The surgeon should be familiar with ALL types of surgical approaches so that he can discuss ALL different options with equal experience. Adult scoliosis is much more challenging to do, so if you have a surgeon who has a practice consisting of exclusively spine surgery, of all age groups, you'll end up with a better-rounded surgeon who is more capable of handling something more complex if a problem arises.

I notice that you will speak directly to your young patients. Can you tell us why you think that is important?

Dr. Mermelstein: The kids are the patients here. They need to take ownership of the decisions, whether they want to or not. Of course, the heavy lifting when it comes to decisions is still done between the parents and myself, but it is very important that the kids feel involved. Otherwise, I might as well be doing veterinary surgery. When the kids have involvement in the decisions, they do not feel as powerless and they are involved in their recovery—and results are better.

What do you recommend to a parent/patient when they don't feel that their medical provider is listening or addressing their concerns?

Dr. Mermelstein: I would ask them if there was another time or forum outside of the traditional office visit where they could communicate. Email has been helpful in getting extra time and answers. Phone conferences after hours are helpful as well. Sometimes the doctor can feel very rushed and strained in the middle of clinic hours. They may be able to listen and respond better in another format. If that doesn't work, you may need to seek answers elsewhere.

Introduction to SEAS

SEAS (Scientific Exercise Approach to Scoliosis) is an Italian-based, conservative exercise treatment based upon scientific research with scoliosis patients.

When asked about the founder, Professor Stefano Negrini, MD, of Milan, Italy explains, "In fact, ISICO (Italian Scientific Spine Institute) was started by my parents, Antonio Negrini and Nevia Verizini, who were both trainers, and my father was also a physiotherapist. I was just the scientist who was so lucky to be born into such a family and to have another clinical master and second professional father, physician Dr. Paolo Sibilla, who taught me the art of both bracing and scoliosis treatment."

Centro Scoliosis Negrini was the foundation for the development of exercises based upon a scientific approach for scoliosis and kyphosis treatment. As the years progressed, their approach improved as the Negrinis exchanged their information and experiences with the top scoliosis centers in six European countries, resulting in a collaborative effort in the study and research of scoliosis.

Professor Negrini, continues the scientific work that his parents began. He and his colleagues study and evaluate new and innovative ways to improve the efficacy of SEAS to achieve optimum results for a scoliotic body.

A Conversation with
Dr. Stefano Negrini

Stefano Negrini, MD, is Scientific Medical Director, as well as one of the founders of ISICO (Italian Scientific Spine Institute) of Milan, Italy. He is the Associate Professor and Director in Physical Medicine and Physiotherapy at the Motor Sciences faculty of University Cattolica del Sacro Cuore in Milan.

After obtaining his degree in medicine, he specialized in Physical and Rehabilitation Medicine. Dr. Negrini has been working on spinal rehabilitation for more than twenty years and is regarded as one of the most influential and respected leaders in Italy on the topic of rehabilitation treatment of scoliosis and other spinal diseases. Dr. Negrini's vast scientific research focuses primarily on evaluating the efficacy of rehabilitation treatment (bracing and exercise) for child and adolescent idiopathic scoliosis, and secondarily on conservative treatment of adult scoliosis, curve evaluation and classification, and lower back and neck pain. Dr. Negrini has received numerous accolades and awards for his research. He is a prolific author who has published over two hundred scientific papers, articles, abstracts, book chapters and textbooks. In addition, he was a founder of the Society on Scoliosis Orthopedic and Rehabilitation Treatment (SOSORT), the international conservative treatment community, where he also has served as Secretary General and President.

You can contact Dr. Negrini or ISICO with further questions at isico@isico.it

Can you explain what type of doctor you are? What is your specific area of expertise?
Dr. Negrini: I'm a physician who specializes only in conservative (non-operative) treatment. In fact, I'm a physiatrist, which is a physical and rehabilitation medicine specialist, and not an orthopedic surgeon. Physical and Rehabilitation Medicine is the specialty which deals with

the management of disabilities. In the area of spinal diseases, we often work on chronic lower back and neck pain, in combination with physical therapists. I strongly believe that we need specific expertise in either surgery or in conservative care. It's not possible today to stay at pace with progress in both of these areas. Orthopedic surgeons specializing in surgery presumably do not have the time to devote to the study of conservative treatment. The more surgical the orthopedic specialty has become, the more surgical were the options indicated for scoliosis patients by orthopedic surgeons.

How would you define Conservative Treatment?

Dr. Negrini: Historically, conservative treatment has been defined by negation, meaning the application of all means other than surgery aimed at avoiding curve progression and potentially improving scoliosis. I prefer the term "rehabilitation treatment," but the term "conservative" is the standard and will remain as such until the various experts in this specialty come together to review the standard of care.

Today, we have evidence as to the efficacy of exercises and braces for scoliosis. We do not have evidence for manual therapy—chiropractic care, osteopathy, or traditional physical therapy modalities. Therefore, the term conservative treatment in the field of scoliosis refers only to exercises and bracing.

Can you describe the SEAS approach?

Dr. Negrini: SEAS principles are based on a specific form of auto-correction, active self-correction, individualized to each patient's scoliosis, and then associated with stabilizing exercises including neuromotor control and proprioceptive training and balance.

Auto-correction is applied to all exercises aimed at reducing the functional impairment typical of scoliosis, and at minimizing the risk of progression.

Which movements are involved in SEAS auto-correction?

Dr. Negrini: These exercises achieve de-rotation (trying to correct the vertebral rotation due to scoliosis), de-flexion (reducing the scoliosis curve(s)), and restoration of the sagittal profile (fighting against the flatback typical of the scoliotic deformity and/or the kyphosis). Treatment is individualized. That is, a patient's specific scoliotic deformity will determine the exercises that are prescribed. Exercises are then adapted and tested for each patient.

What is the main goal of SEAS exercises?

Dr. Negrini: The goal of the exercises is training motor behavior, self-awareness, and reflex responses. This is what has been shown to be useful in our scoliosis patients. As much as possible, we use the active auto-correction. Other conservative methods may use physical aids throughout the course of treatment. SEAS only use aids at the beginning in order to speed up learning. Auto-correction is learned gradually over time. Like learning to dance, it takes practice. You cannot do it correctly immediately, and so we use some external aids during this learning phase.

How many patients do you treat per year?

Dr. Negrini: I personally treat more than one thousand patients conservatively per year. I see each patient every four to six months for twenty- to thirty-minute evaluations. At this time, I not only evaluate, but also motivate patients to be compliant with their therapy and bracing. Treating conservatively less than three hundred patients per year, according to the SOSORT (www.sosort.org) criteria for brace treatment management, is not enough for specific expertise in this area.

At what curve degree do you begin the SEAS?

Dr. Negrini: On the average, we start at 15°. The first step is observation. Then, in an effort to avoid bracing, we start SEAS exercises as soon as we see significant risk factors for progression—such as curves greater than 15° or less than 15° with a significant hump or a flatback, a positive family history, or if the patient is in a rapid growth period. Conversely, if a person has reached physical maturity or has an insignificant hump with a curve higher than 15°, we can choose not to take any action. For us, decisions always come from many factors, not only Cobb (curve) degrees. If there are no other risk factors, we may not start at all. The process is fully personalized.

How often do you change a patient's exercise regime?
Dr. Negrini: Exercises are modified on a regular basis every two to three months, according to the patient's growth, individual capacities, what has been learned, and so on. We adapt the exercises to what the patient is able to do and, consequently, the idea of "perfection" changes over time.

SEAS database consists of more than a thousand exercises which continue to be changed and adapted as we learn what is most effective. We also accept the idea that exercises will change completely according to new scientific discoveries. In this respect, SEAS is not a method but an approach. It is not closed nor fully codified. As we have changed in the past, we are sure we will change again as new knowledge becomes available from both our own research, as well as from colleagues worldwide.

As the result of a project we are running, this exercise database (www.scoliosismanager.com) is now accessible to patients around the world. However, it is important to remember that for the management of scoliosis, these exercises must include active self-correction to be effective. (Authors' note: patients should not select exercises on their own without a health provider's diagnosis and advice.)

Do children who have successfully finished their bracing need to maintain an exercise program to prevent further curve progression?
Dr. Negrini: No. Treatment must start and finish. Scoliosis patients need a healthy behavior like any other adult to maintain good physical fitness, which will definitely help their backs. If, however, the scoliosis progresses, we would need to restore specific exercises in order to try and avoid surgery.

BRACING

What is the role of bracing?
Dr. Negrini: Exercises will never be as efficacious as bracing because of the importance of external pushes provided by the brace. In fact, auto-correction achieved through exercises several minutes a day will never be the same as the correction that can be maintained when using a brace throughout the day.

The standard of care for bracing in the U.S. is when a child's curve reaches 25°. When do you begin bracing?
Dr. Negrini: Rigid bracing begins between 25° to 30°. We begin bracing with the soft braces (SpineCor®) between 20° and 30°. Again, the decision to brace is determined by many factors.

In the U.S., bracing varies from sixteen hours to twenty-three hours a day. How many hours do you recommend your patients brace per day?
Dr. Negrini: Rigid braces can be prescribed eighteen to twenty-three hours per day according to individual need. In our view, it all depends on balancing two factors: the fewer hours, the better for the patient; but the fewer hours, the more possible a scoliosis progression. Our first aim is to reduce the burden on the patient, but this all depends on the scoliosis curve. If you are facing a scoliosis that can be compared to a very unfriendly cat, you can take it carefully in your hands, but if you are facing a scoliosis-*tiger* all you can do is to erect walls around her.

The factors we consider in order to make the most informed choice include: Cobb degrees, physical structure of patient (thin or strong), the period of growth (rapid or slow), bone age (young or mature), and risk for progression (high versus low). All these elements will help us determine the amount of hours we recommend our patient to brace. When you use a more rigid brace, sometimes you can reduce the hours worn. However, this is not so simplistic since a very deformed spine needs to grow as much as possible in a correct position, which requires more hours of bracing per day.

Brace compliance is a big issue with teens. Can you tell us about your approach to both brace and exercise compliance?
Dr. Negrini: In my view, and that of SOSORT, obtaining compliance is mostly how the treating team approaches the patient. It is not just what you say to a patient but how you say it. We presented a SOSORT abstract in Barcelona that won the SOSORT Award and is published in Scoliosis Journal (www.scoliosisjournal.com), showing the highest compliance rates ever published: an average of almost 90 percent. This means that patients could be made to be compliant to bracing. If you want an asymptomatic teenager to wear plastic for

years, you must believe in what you are doing, and you must apply all possible techniques to reinforce your message.

What type of brace do you prefer to use?

Dr. Negrini: The two main rigid braces we use are the Sibilla Brace and the Sforzesco Brace (www.scoliosisjournal.com/content/6/1/8). Our braces are custom-made following a cast mold or a CAD/CAM construction after laser body scanning. While the construction is similar in both, the Sibilla is made of a less rigid material. We fully comply with the SOSORT guidelines for management of bracing which, in our view, is mandatory to obtain good results. I suggest all the readers look at these guidelines available at www.scoliosisjournal. com/content/4/1/2.

Literature has indicated that bracing over 40° is not effective. Do you continue to brace your patient if their curve is over 40°?

Dr. Negrini: Yes. Surgery for scoliosis is fusing the spine, which means losing one of its functions—movement, in favor of another—stability. A patient with a 40° curve has a cosmetic deformity, nothing else. Generally, they don't have any other symptoms and vital capacity is not usually compromised at this level. In Italy, we would view surgery as preventative. We can accept such prevention only in really extreme cases when the hope of stability into adulthood is completely lost. To me, we have to first try conservative treatment to reduce the deformity as much as possible. What we can guarantee with good bracing is an aesthetic result (www.scoliosisjournal.com/content/4/1/18) and in curves between 45° and 55° to 60° we have an 8° to 10° curve reduction on average (The Spine Journal 2011: abstract presented in Lyon SOSORT Meeting/www.scoliosisjournal.com/content/4/S2/O50). This means that some patients remain stable or progress a little, but others "win the jackpot" and reduce their curve over 15° to 20°. In the case of large, progressive curves, surgery must be considered. But in the case of curves that respond to bracing, surgery is usually avoided.

Our approach to these high degree curves is to ask the patient and family what they want to do. If they want to try conservative treatment, which is what we suggest, we have six months to see what can be achieved. If we are not able to achieve the outcome that the team desires, we tell the patient and family to consult with a surgeon in order to make an informed decision.

In the U.S., the brace prescribed most frequently is the Boston Brace. What is your opinion on the effectiveness of this brace?

Dr. Negrini: While the Boston Brace is an effective brace, I use other braces for three main reasons. First, posterior is where we have to push more, and I prefer that here we have more rigidity. Second, compliance is important to successful bracing and front opening braces are easier for the patient to manage. And finally, the Boston Brace has a problem in treating thoracic curves. We need a higher profile brace than the classic Boston Brace to treat the thoracic curves. In our braces, we have an anterior closure over the breasts to give more rigidity to the thoracic pushes. With this we can reach curves with the highest apex up to vertebra T5, which is more than what is reported with other braces in the literature. Above T5 apex, we help the underarm brace by adding a cervical push (not really a collar, something less obvious that goes under the clothes).

Do you recommend the use of a nighttime brace? If so, then under what circumstances?

Dr. Negrini: I do not recommend a nighttime brace, because I don't think it can give real advantages with respect to exercises. There is a paper showing superiority of the Providence Brace (nighttime) with respect to the Wilmington Brace (daytime). This is astonishing to me since with a well-made brace, the more you use it the better the results you would have. The literature is quite clear that the brace is useful if used full-time, meaning twenty hours per day or more. Nighttime bracing can be useful in low degree curves when you do not have a more physiology-based approach like exercises, or even like an elastic brace.

BRACE WEANING

Some doctors take up to six months for their patients to be weaned from their brace. What is your protocol for brace weaning?

Dr. Negrini: In my view, the neuromotor system cannot react adequately to maintain the correction in six months. This could be good if you think of scoliosis only as a bone deformity. But when you recognize (as it is written in the literature) that there is also a postural component based on muscles and reaction to gravity force, you give time to this system to react adequately, which in the end, will give better results. When good bone maturity is reached (Risser 3-4), we start going under eighteen hours per day, which usually takes another twenty-four to thirty months before the brace is completely eliminated. In fact, the patients reduce the wearing time two hours every six months. So, gradually we reach the point when the ring apophysis (a measurement indicating that the spine is fully mature) usually closes at Risser 5. To avoid losing the correction, a gradual weaning is done in conjunction with exercises. This could explain why at the end of treatment, on average, we have an 8° to 9° curve reduction while others usually do not have improvements. We do not lose correction while weaning (and this has been proven in another paper we published: www.scoliosisjournal.com/content/4/1/8).

SCOLISCORE®

Will the new ScoliScore® saliva test change the way you treat your patients?

Dr. Negrini: Perhaps. I don't know. The history of scoliosis treatment has been full of promising treatments/evaluations that, in the long run, failed (i.e., electrical stimulation). The most important goal is avoiding the risk of problems in adulthood, stabilizing curves at less than 30 Cobb degrees, and preventing aesthetic problems. I am very cautious in all individual cases when deciding what to do, even in the face of any promising new test.

What can cause a skeletally matured person's 30° curve to progress another 10° in less than a year post-bracing?

Dr. Negrini: I've had three cases that progressed rapidly after weaning from their brace at skeletal maturity. Consequently, these patients were treated with SEAS exercises and recovered completely, achieving better results than seen at the end of brace treatment. One case has been published in Scoliosis Journal (www.scoliosisjournal.com/content/3/1/20). During brace treatment, these patients performed improper exercises. Our hypothesis is that their neuromotor control system had not been able to adapt properly during the weaning phase. My interpretation of this phenomenon (www.scoliosisjournal.com/content/3/1/20) is that the neuromotor system did not behave properly, as the brace interfered with its development and, therefore, had to be re-trained.

SURGERY

When might you recommend surgery for a person with scoliosis?

Dr. Negrini: I recommend surgery when problems are guaranteed into adulthood. This is an individual choice depending on Cobb degrees and many other factors. All patients must be well aware of risks on both sides, fusion versus conservative treatment for the rest of their life. Min Mehta, one of the most famous physicians dealing with scoliosis, never had her curve operated on and it was around 90°. Therefore, any individual choice is possible.

I think of how I would advise my own daughter if she had a large, significant thoracic curve with no other problems. If her curve was over 55° before starting any treatment, I would carefully discuss the possibility of fusion surgery because according to our study results, it is highly improbable that she could reduce her curve below 45°. Following some months of treatment without significant results, I would strongly suggest surgery, or I would suggest surgery immediately if she was not a candidate for bracing and her curve was above 55° to 60°. The final decision is made on a case-by-case basis, such as when occurring with a lumbar curve, which can be more dangerous and must be reduced. Or there may be other problems like significant imbalances, flatback, and so on that may require a surgical solution. All these factors must be taken into account with patients, their parents, and the multidisciplinary care team.

What are your guidelines when recommending surgery on a skeletally mature patient?
Dr. Negrini: To me, an adult scoliosis should only be operated on if they have significant symptoms, such as a scoliosis that is not stable (i.e., progressive), and specific exercises fail to stabilize it. Moreover, surgery should be considered when, despite conservative treatment, problems persist, such as persistent pain, impaired quality of life, diminished lung capacity, or a significant imbalance. It must be clear to adult patients that if exercises succeed in stabilizing their curves, they must exercise for the rest of their life. If they cannot accept this, then surgery is preferable.

Introduction to the Schroth Method

The Schroth Method originated in Germany with Katharina Schroth, who suffered both physically and emotionally from her scoliosis deformity. Born in 1894, the best treatment available for scoliosis at the time was bracing. By the early 1900s, posterior fusion surgery was beginning to be performed. Though she wore a brace as a young woman, Katharina's ultimate goal was to be able to live without a brace and to have straight posture with no obvious deformity. Inspired one day by looking at a half-deflated ball, she couldn't help but notice that when inflated with air, the flattened part of the ball became round and firm again. This observation led her to think of the possibility of changing her own body using the same concept. With the use of multiple mirrors, she worked very hard at first to correct any postural collapse and then further opening her concavities with a breathing technique she developed, called rotational breathing. With continued practice Katharina eventually witnessed a consistent change in her own scoliotic body. This successful experiment was the genesis of the Schroth Method. By 1921, Katharina Schroth had received training in physiology and physical therapy, established her own clinic and dedicated the rest of her life to helping thousands of people with their spinal deformities.

Katharina's daughter, Christa Lehnert-Schroth also became formally trained in Germany as a physical therapist. Mother and daughter successfully developed their spinal deformity inpatient program in Bad Sobernheim, Germany. Their clinic grew to serve more than 1200 patients annually. In 1995, the clinic was sold to the Asklepios Hospital Group. Historically, patients were seen for intensive inpatient treatment for four-to-six weeks. Today, there is more variation in treatment visits.

Elena Salva, PT, brought the Schroth Method to her clinic in Spain in the 1960s. Today, Manuel Rigo, MD, and his wife, Gloria

Quera-Salva, DO, run the Clinic. Dr. Rigo has taught the Schroth Method to physical therapists since the late 1980s. In 2009, he formalized his own training program with the blessing of Ms. Lehnert-Schroth. The Barcelona Physiotherapy School (BSPTS) adheres to the original techniques of Katharina Schroth and Christa Lehnert-Schroth.

In 2003, U.S. physical therapist Beth Janssen traveled to Barcelona, Spain, where she was trained and certified by Dr. Manuel Rigo in the Schroth Method. Her passion to find an alternative to the "wait-and-see" approach was fueled when her own son was diagnosed with scoliosis. In 2006, Beth, along with her business partner, Rhonda Campo, opened the first physical therapy clinics in the United States dedicated to the treatment of scoliosis using the Schroth Method—Scoliosis Rehab in Stevens Point, Wisconsin and Phoenix, Arizona.

The Schroth Method Comes to the United States

A Conversation with
Beth Janssen and Rhonda Campo

Beth Janssen, PT, co-founder of Scoliosis Rehab has been a practicing physical therapist since 1986, when she graduated from the Mayo School of Health Related Sciences in Rochester, MN. She has worked extensively in hospital settings, where her practice focused on evaluation and treatment of spinal and TMJ dysfunction, women's health problems, scoliosis rehabilitation, and mentoring of new physical therapists. She has done advanced studies in the McKenzie approach to treating spinal dysfunction, along with Muscle Energy Techniques and Myofascial Release training.

Beth developed a special interest in scoliosis after her son was diagnosed with scoliosis. She trained in Spain in the conservative care of scoliosis with Dr. Manuel Rigo, developer of the Rigo System Cheneau® brace, and world-renowned expert in the Schroth Method for conservative care of scoliosis. She is one of the first certified Schroth therapists in the United States and has assisted Dr. Rigo in all courses for physical therapists in the U.S. since 2004.

Rhonda Campo, BSE, MBA, co-founder of Scoliosis Rehab, completed her undergraduate work at the University of Pennsylvania where she focused on bioengineering and economics. She received her MBA from the Wharton School with distinction in health care finance. As a Heinz Fellow at Carnegie-Mellon University, she completed her PhD coursework in Health Economics and Public Policy. She has been a Kellogg Foundation Health Policy Fellow at HCFA, Director of Finance at one of the Harvard hospitals, an investment banker specializing in healthcare and biotech, and COO at the former AMSCO International.

Ms. Campo resides in Columbus, Ohio with her family and spends her time on community service, consulting, and studying scoliosis from various perspectives.

How did you learn about the Schroth Method?

Ms. Janssen: When my son was diagnosed with scoliosis I didn't think I could passively "watch and wait" to see if his condition deteriorated. So I began researching other treatments for scoliosis. I learned about the Schroth Method when I read Martha Hawes' book, *Scoliosis and the Human Spine.* In this book, she mentions an exercise model, the Schroth Method, which has been used successfully in Germany for over ninety years. After reading her book, I called Germany to see if I could attend the Asklepios Schroth clinic with my son. They sent me to Dr. Rigo in Spain, where the patients were taught in English.

In October of 2003, I traveled to Barcelona, Spain with my son. Dr. Rigo trained and certified me in the Schroth Method while I was there. I returned to the U.S. as one of the first physical therapists to be trained in the Schroth Method.

Having seen the benefits of Schroth therapy, I was passionate about utilizing the techniques in the job I held at a local hospital. But most hospital physical therapy departments don't specialize in a single type of patient. So I began to think that other physical therapists in the U.S. needed to learn about Schroth when they treated a spinal patient.

At my request, in 2005, Dr. Rigo did the first training course in the U.S. for physical therapists in Stevens Point, Wisconsin. I was the clinical assistant for this ten-day course, which certified several other physical therapists here.

What led to the opening of Scoliosis Rehab?

Ms. Janssen: Two weeks before Dr. Rigo came to the U.S. for that training course, a woman in Pennsylvania, Rhonda Campo, came across a story in a Wisconsin newspaper about my Barcelona study and certification.

What she didn't know, of course, was that I still needed demonstration patients for Dr. Rigo to use during his course. Fortunately, Rhonda had already read about the Schroth Method and spoken with Martha Hawes, so she agreed to come and bring her two scoliotic children to Wisconsin as training cases for Dr. Rigo.

We were both impressed with Dr. Rigo's knowledge, as well as the physical and psychological impact of Schroth training on our families.

And, we were like-minded that this treatment should be available to parents, children, and physicians in the U.S.

Normally, physical therapy clinics do not specialize in a particular disorder. But in 2006, we opened Scoliosis Rehab, Inc. in Stevens Point, WI. We were the first physical therapy clinic in the U.S. dedicated to the treatment of scoliosis and other spinal deformities. Moreover, we realized in order to really excel at Schroth-based physical therapy, you need to consistently treat a variety of spine patients.

In 2009, with Dr. Rigo's blessing and following further training in Barcelona, we began to certify physical therapists ourselves at Scoliosis Rehab, Inc. To date, we have taught over fifty U.S., Australian, and Malaysian physical therapists.

We have a list of trained and certified Schroth physical therapists on our web site, www.scoliosisrehab.com.

How does the Schroth Method work?

Ms. Janssen: The Schroth Method uses specific exercises based on an individual's curve pattern. This method is based on sensorimotor and kinesthetic principles. That means that patients have to develop a self-awareness of where their bodies are in space, how they hold their bodies now, and how they should actually be holding their bodies.

The patient learns the corrected posture by actually practicing moving the body through space and holding this reformed position. The physical therapist works with the patient to help develop this self-awareness in three dimensions. The Schroth-based treatment uses exercises to correct the scoliotic posture with proprioceptive and external stimulation and mirrors.

Proprioceptive stimulation means that you have to perceive where your body is in space, relative to the other parts of your body, and be aware of the effort needed to move the body into the more balanced alignment. The external stimulation is initially the hands of a well-trained physical therapist guiding the treatment, and also the pads and props used by the therapist. Eventually, as deeper self-awareness is developed, the patient can find the corrected position independently and maintain it at least partially in daily life.

The patients use an individually-developed routine of corrections to lift themselves out of the curve pattern in three dimensions, along with a new breathing pattern to further expand concave or collapsed areas.

With these exercises, we are correcting as much of the postural collapse as possible, in order to decrease the mechanical forces that may be contributing to the progression of the curve. The goal is to learn the new corrected position so completely that the patient automatically maintains this corrected posture to some degree as they go through activities of daily life. A patient with scoliosis finds it most comfortable to stand in a posture that reinforces the scoliosis curvatures.

The goal for a Schroth patient trained to stand in a non-scoliotic posture, will hopefully, with practice, be able to subconsciously assume the corrected posture rather than the collapsed scoliotic posture throughout their life. We believe that will result in a permanently better back health for the patient.

When can a person begin to see a change?

Ms. Janssen: As far as a person noticing a change, this varies depending on the individual. Most people with myofascial pain will feel a positive change within a short period of time. If there are some secondary problems, such as arthritic changes, or disc issues combined with pressure on the nerves, the exercises may not ameliorate the pain.

Most adolescents will see changes in the shape of their torso within the first week of training. This positive change will happen when the patient does the muscle activation. Once a person sinks back into their old posture, the change will be gone. The longer the patient remains in the corrected posture, the easier it becomes to find the corrected posture and stay there.

With the Schroth exercises, the physical therapist is trying to teach patients a new way to hold themselves in three dimensions. We work to have the patient recognize what the corrected position feels like and then to know how to stabilize the body in this new position.

What is the routine when a new patient arrives at your clinic?

Ms. Campo: For patients arriving at our clinic in Stevens Point, WI, or Phoenix, AZ, we follow a standard routine. First, a physical therapist that has advanced certification in the Schroth-based method from the BSPTS does a comprehensive physical therapy evaluation and history. X-ray films are reviewed with the patient to ascertain Cobb angles and rotation, and the curve pattern is categorized according to the Rigo Classification.

The therapist then proceeds to educate the patient and their parent on anatomy, the three-dimensional nature of scoliosis, individual posture, body mechanics, and the vicious cycle that will worsen the patient's posture if left unchecked.

Once the patient has a sense of what their spines look like and how that causes them to hold their body, walk, sit, etc., our physical therapist moves onto teaching specific beginning exercises.

This is a very interactive process in which the patient learns an exercise, the physical therapist watches the exercise and modifies it based on examination of the patient, and then the patient performs the exercise again. Once each exercise is well understood and performed independently, the patient will then be taught additional exercises based on their own abilities and needs.

Proper breathing techniques are a large component of each exercise. When patients are proficient with their own exercises, the therapist begins to teach them how to incorporate the corrections into everyday activities.

Is there a minimum age requirement to learn this method of exercise?
Ms. Janssen: We follow the guidelines of Dr. Rigo from BSPTS. This recommendation includes waiting until the child is ten years old for girls and twelve years old for boys. Since girls enter their pubertal growth spurt before boys, we want to give them the information that they need when they are actively growing. Committing to the Schroth exercises requires a certain level of developmental maturity in order to be able to focus on posture and alignment.

Does your curve have to be a certain degree before treatment can begin?
Ms. Janssen: So as not to over-treat, we usually begin the exercises at a 15° Cobb angle, based on the chance of progression. If there is any pain or other problem present, we may begin at a greater or lesser Cobb

angle. Also, if there is a strong family history of scoliosis, we may recommend bracing or exercise earlier than we would when there is no history.

Can the Schroth Method benefit fused patients?

Ms. Janssen: We believe it is important for a surgically-fused individual to understand where their bodies are in space: Is the pelvis out of balance to one side? Are the shoulders level over the rib cage? Are the shoulders level or is there some collapse? Is the head tilted?

Patients who have had surgery should learn about symmetry and balance, strategies for stretching, if needed, and core stabilization strengthening with good alignment, while using the exercises and breath to expand the collapsed areas of the trunk. The physical therapist must always be mindful of the fusion, as the patient should not be doing any aggressive stretches.

It's also essential to consider the "wear and tear" at the ends of the fused site. All the movement that would have been distributed throughout the spine now occurs above and below the fusion only. We also believe low impact activities with the spine in neutral will prolong the health of the post-surgical back. In some ways, it is even more important for a person with a fusion to understand how to take care of their back.

Are exercises learned one-on-one or are the children seen in a group?

Ms. Campo: A physical therapist, certified in the method, teaches the therapeutic exercises one-on-one. Most of the time, in the U.S., the exercises are taught individually, because the patient's spinal curve, rotation, degree of trunk imbalance, and muscle condition is unique. This way, we are able to tailor the exercises to each patient's specific needs.

When a patient comes for an intensive one- to two-week session, we offer them some time to practice their exercises in what we refer to as "Open Gym." During Open Gym, the patients gather in front of their wall-bars with no screens separating them from other patients. Each patient concentrates on practicing their specific exercises, but can chat with the other patients and a therapist who oversees the Open Gym.

In addition, we do have some special sessions during the year where we offer group instruction for adolescent girls, for example, or for post-menopausal women, who have been trained at the clinic but want a refresher.

Open Gym and group sessions have an added psychosocial benefit of providing emotional support by others facing the same condition and issues. People who meet under these circumstances frequently tell us that they no longer feel so isolated or unusual because they've met someone who can relate to their situation.

Is there any pain or discomfort when first learning to do these exercises?
Ms. Janssen: There should be no pain with the treatment. Sometimes there is stretching of soft tissue and/or muscle fatigue, which may result from the patient working the muscles in a new way. If a patient experiences any pain, they need to tell the therapist, so that the exercises can be adjusted.

Most adolescents can perform the exercises with a relatively brief period of rest between sessions. The adolescents will be tired after their appointment, but generally not sore.

As with any activity, aging must be taken into account. Our adult population consists of people of all ages including post-menopausal women. We frequently adjust their treatment plans to provide more time between appointments, so that these women can allow their bodies to acclimate to new movement patterns and tissue stimulation.

In your opinion, why do you believe there is a different approach to the treatment of scoliosis in the U.S. versus Europe?
Ms. Campo: This is a very complicated issue and multi-determined. Historically, scoliosis has been treated with exercises for at least 4,000 years. Viable surgical treatments, on the other hand, have only been available since the early 1900s.

There is a rich history of country-specific exercises in Europe, the Middle East, and Japan. Medical providers in these countries grow up with, and are trained in, these conservative methods. The European concept and model of using exercise has been developed with different methods evolving in each country. In addition, surgery is not as widely available in many European countries as a result of their government-controlled healthcare reimbursement.

The United States, on the other hand, does not have a long history of physical therapy in relation to scoliosis. Physical therapy exercises were briefly tried from the 1930s to the 1950s, but were not specific to curve patterns. At the same time, surgical methods were being improved. In the U.S., the history of surgical treatment for scoliosis actually may be longer than the history of physical therapy for scoliosis.[1] We believe that the efficacy of therapeutic exercise as a way of impacting the lives of people with scoliosis in the U.S. has never been adequately studied. Most physicians, other medical providers, and even physical therapists, are not taught about exercises for scoliosis during their training.

In both Europe and the United States, you will find some physicians who are interested in using specific exercises in the treatment of scoliosis. Martha Hawes, in her book, *Scoliosis and the Human Spine*, explains why U.S. medical practitioners have treated scoliosis patients primarily with surgery. Part of the problem accounting for the lack of support for using exercises to treat scoliosis in the U.S. may be the historical lack of "Randomized Controlled Trials" (RCT) in studies showing that these exercises can work. This is because RCT can be impractical, unethical, and expensive to complete.

Historically, there has not been grant funding to support this type of research. Physical therapists do not learn about exercises for scoliosis during their education, so those therapists who go on to complete their doctorate degrees have not generally been aware of the research opportunity exploring exercise for scoliosis.

Medical costs also play a role in determining what treatment is offered. European countries with socialized medical models offer a continuum of care that begins with the cheapest therapies, which also tend to be the least technologically sophisticated therapies; thus, exercise and bracing would be prescribed before surgery.

Conversely, in the U.S., patients have been free to go to the physician of their choice. So if a patient goes to an orthopedic surgeon for scoliosis before going to a physical therapist or rehabilitative medicine doctor, it is more likely that surgery will be prescribed rather than a conservative exercise treatment.

Surgical training in the U.S. does not currently include a non-surgical rotation, so most surgeons are not even aware of other options for scoliosis treatment. Additionally, private insurance and the availability of philanthropic institutions, such as the Shriners Hospital system, which provides no-cost care for those who cannot afford to pay, make surgery much more available for Americans.

Finally, there are those in our fast-paced society who would rather have the intense surgical experience and take six weeks or so to recover than spend twenty-plus hours in a brace each day until skeletally mature, and then twenty minutes per day on exercises for the rest of their life. Other cultures, in general, have more of a long-term wellness focus.

Whether in Europe, Asia, the Middle East, or the U.S., it's important that the treatment of scoliosis be seen as a continuum. Some patients, who progress to surgery after trying exercises and bracing, report having a more positive experience overall. Conservative treatment for patients and family should begin with an explanation of the continuum of care. In addition, patient education should include posture, body mechanics, and nutrition for a lifetime of healthy bones.

The creation of SOSORT in 2004 has helped to bring together international clinicians and scientists interested in the conservative management of scoliosis, giving them an opportunity to share their knowledge. The goal is to have a positive impact on research and treatment worldwide. Surgeons and non-surgical specialists are beginning to dialogue with each other.

Scoliosis care must be viewed as a continuum and those who advocate conservative management need to see the limits of their treatments, just as surgeons need to see the limits of theirs.

The best outcomes occur when patients are followed by a multidisciplinary team (e.g., orthopedic surgeon, physical therapist, orthotist). But even with the best conservative care, sometimes surgery is necessary. My own daughter progressed to surgery despite exemplary brace and exercise compliance. She was fortunate to have only a selective fusion, as the result of a team of professionals thinking about the best outcome for the whole patient rather than simply their own area of expertise. In addition, her recovery was rapid as a result of understanding her body mechanics and having well-developed supporting musculature prior to the surgery.

SOSORT has produced a very helpful paper outlining how treatment should progress as the curve progresses.[2] Hopefully, the U.S. will adopt this team approach used in much of the rest of the world.

Why aren't there any randomized controlled clinical trials for the Schroth Method?

Ms. Campo: There is a joke among healthcare researchers that goes something like this: A researcher is writing a grant to explore a new drug that holds great promise. First, the study design has to be reviewed by epidemiologists to make sure that there could be no catastrophic unintended results. Then, the biostatisticians get involved to determine how many and what types of patients would have to be recruited for the study. Next, accountants need to review the funding request to make sure that that researcher is asking for enough money to properly conduct the study and cover the university's costs.

The Institutional Review Board is perhaps the toughest step, as this panel needs to review the entire protocol and ensure that no harm could come to any patient who participates in the study. The young researcher is then ready to send her grant off to Washington in order for a federal agency to review it and determine if the grant is worthy of funding. But first, she needs to take an aspirin for the massive headache that designing and writing the study has caused. An older and wiser colleague gives her an aspirin and reminds the young researcher of a very sad fact—if aspirin had to be studied in a randomized controlled trial today, it would never make it past all of the regulators!

The Harrington rods and spinal surgery were developed at a time when regulations around medical research were much more lax than today. Just as it would most likely be impractical and unethical to perform a randomized controlled clinical trial of scoliosis surgery, so it is with physical therapy for scoliosis. Which child gets to learn the physical therapy exercises? Which child doesn't? Who decides?

In addition, there is some selection bias in which patients (and parents of patients) want to try physical therapy. Physical therapy requires daily discipline and scheduling, which is not something that every teenager is prepared for or wants to do. Again, would it be ethical to select a child for a physical therapy trial when the child and parents know that that child does not want to follow-through with exercise for the rest of their life?

Hopefully, there will be a body of case studies that begin to evaluate outcomes of physical therapy for scoliosis. In addition, descriptive studies may help us to understand the characteristics of patients and curve patterns that respond positively to physical therapy. Outside the U.S., there are already some valid studies to be found in reputable, peer-reviewed journals.

Are there any exercises that are not healthy for a scoliotic spine?
Ms. Janssen: We advocate exercises for people with scoliosis to be performed with the spine in neutral. With idiopathic scoliosis, the vertebral bodies of the main curve become wedge-shaped—each vertebra is taller in the front than the back, and taller on the convex (rib hump or lumbar prominence) side of the curve than on the concave side. There is also usually some collapse in the concave areas.

When people with scoliosis bend forward, the prominences become more noticeable. This flexion causes increased torsion in the spine, which then pushes the spine more into the pattern of the scoliosis. The wedge shape of the thoracic vertebrae can lead to loss of thoracic kyphosis, which is a loss of the normal shape of the spine when viewed from the side. In some people with scoliosis, the thoracic spine can actually become flat or go into lordosis (an inward curve of the spine when looking at the side view). So when a person with scoliosis does backward bending (or extension), they push the spine forward, which exaggerates the forward push on the thoracic spine causing a reduction in thoracic kyphosis. We want a certain amount of kyphosis in the thoracic spine because this allows room for the heart and lungs and more normal alignment of other spinal structures.

Just as flexion and extension increase the magnitude of the front and back planes of the curve(s), side bending increases the size of the lateral curve(s). In scoliosis, one curve doesn't generally exist alone; most often there is at least a small compensatory curve above or below the primary curve. We teach that all daily movements and exercises are to be performed with the spine in neutral in 3D with self-elongation.

We do not advocate side bending or rotational exercises, because when you move into side bending or rotation, you will be straightening one curve but feeding into the other curve.

Is there an impact on curves when doing push-ups and crunches?
Ms. Janssen: Push-ups are fine as long as the person can keep their trunk in neutral. We advocate that all exercises be done with the spine in neutral as described above. We have other abdominal exercises that we teach instead of crunches, which can strengthen the abdominals without feeding into the pattern of the scoliosis.

What does it mean to keep your spine in neutral?
Ms. Janssen: Spinal neutral means holding the back in a position where from the side view you have the normal curves of the back, an inward curve at the neck and low back (which is called lordosis), and an outward curve (or kyphosis) at the rib cage. It also means that the pelvis is balanced in a left-to-right position and that it is not rotated. This is something that we teach in therapy.

A person should try to keep the back more or less straight with a small inward curve in the low back without twisting or side bending. This neutral posture should be the goal during all activities of daily living. Because people with scoliosis do not feel like they are standing in an uneven posture, learning to stand and sit in neutral requires repeated effort.

What about participation in exercise programs such as yoga and Pilates?
Ms. Campo: Yoga and Pilates and Schroth do not have to be mutually exclusive; in fact, there are similarities between the Schroth exercises and some yoga and Pilates techniques. For a patient who is interested, we would caution them to seek out an instructor who understands

the complexity of scoliosis and other spinal conditions, or have their Schroth therapist work with them to modify their yoga and Pilates' stances. One of the advantages of the Schroth Method is that none of the movements put any part of the back at risk.

What are some of the benefits yoga and Pilates can offer to a person with scoliosis?

Ms. Campo: Focusing on the breath is one aspect of yoga and Pilates that is excellent for spine patients. The breathing techniques are quite similar to the rotational breathing taught in Schroth. Yoga and Pilates are very effective at teaching patients self-awareness of their breath mechanics.

When the patient has properly elongated the spine, as taught by Schroth techniques, the breathing mechanics of yoga and Pilates have their greatest impact. Also, the stabilizing, mobilizing, and strengthening of the body via yoga and Pilates are great for a scoliotic patient. However, when scoliosis or another spine dysfunction is present, mobilizing the body in a flexing/rotating or side bending position will not be beneficial.

Can you explain the differences between yoga and Pilates and the Schroth exercises?

Ms. Janssen: Schroth therapists favor exercises that promote self-elongation, keep the spine in neutral in three dimensions, and have been selected based on an evaluation of each individual's curve pattern.

We cannot support exercises that move the spine out of a neutral position for several reasons. Foremost is the anatomical fact that scoliosis is a three-dimensional problem. In scoliosis, groups of adjacent vertebrae form a torsion region (i.e., the vertebrae are twisted and compressed together) with the vertebrae moving relatively forward and translating and rotating to the same side.

Bear in mind, this region is joined by transitional regions to the next curve above or below. When you bend forward, called "flexion," disc pressure is increased at the bend, but more so when the bend occurs at the transitional vertebrae between curves. Likewise, backwards bending, called "extension" pushes those vertebrae, which have already moved forward, further forward.

Secondly, since one curve doesn't generally exist alone, there is usually a compensating curve that tries to mirror the primary curve. Therefore, an instructor must be aware that when "untwisting" one curve with an exercise, they are actually increasing the twist of another curve. The same is true for yoga stances that include side bending.

When a strong believer in yoga or Pilates disagrees with a Schroth Method advocate, they may say, "But what's the difference, we're mobilizing the spine and so is the Schroth Method." The difference is that the Schroth exercises include positions that never increase the disc pressure, focus on lengthening and elongating without twisting the spine, and teach core strengthening while maintaining a neutral, de-rotated spinal position.

In the Schroth method, there is only one exercise that does include minimal side bending, and that is the advanced Pendulum exercise, which is performed with the patient completely elongated so as to produce an insignificant amount of closing of the curves.

In addition, many people with scoliosis are more hyper-mobile, or experience greater joint laxity, than those without scoliosis, so flexibility exercises should be used with caution, always following a careful history and analysis of the patient's specific physical condition.

What exercises can you recommend?
Ms. Janssen: Low impact aerobic exercises such as walking, biking, and elliptical training are acceptable. If you enjoy running, do it in moderation and never when you are tired. Keep in mind that people with scoliosis need to be able to elongate and stand tall with muscle activation to prevent the collapse of the concave areas when performing these activities.

Most importantly, being aware how you move your spine when performing any exercise is essential. Also, when your body becomes fatigued, the natural tendency is to slump back into the scoliotic posture. The patient should exercise when well-rested and proper posture can be maintained.

Does this method require full-time bracing in conjunction with the exercises?

Ms. Janssen: We advocate part-time or full-time bracing for adolescents based on magnitude of the Cobb angle, skeletal maturity, and risk of progression from other known factors, such as family history. The decision to brace is made on a case-by-case basis, ideally by a multidisciplinary team.

Are there any studies that show that this type of treatment is more effective than full-time bracing alone?

Ms. Campo: These specific exercises are designed to be used with or without bracing, depending on the skeletal maturity of the patient and some other factors. If the person is skeletally immature and the Cobb angle is greater than 25°, the exercises should be used in conjunction with a good brace from a reputable orthotist. Once the person is skeletally mature, that individual would be weaned from the brace and continue with the exercises. There are some studies that look at the use of exercises and how it may affect the curve.[3,4] However, it is important to note that some curves will not be stabilized with just exercises and bracing, and will require surgery.

The Schroth Method also encourages a Cheneau TLSO with Rigo modifications for a brace. Why and how is it different from other TLSO braces?

Ms. Janssen: A Cheneau TLSO with Rigo modifications is a three-dimensional brace that is not full-contact. This means it does not touch the torso everywhere as it wraps around the person.

This brace reinforces the correction that the person learns in their exercises. The brace puts pressures on the prominences on the patient's back (e.g., the rib hump) and sides, as well as on the prominent parts of the rib cage. The brace has "rooms," or open spaces, built in the front of the prominences and the back over the concave areas, thus, encouraging the patient to breathe into the open space. In this way, the brace becomes dynamic when the person is trained to breathe appropriately. Performed with the exercises, the breathing pattern is called rotational breathing.

Once the person learns to hold the body in the best position, this breathing is then used to further expand the concave areas. If the patient were placed in either a full-contact TLSO or a "soft" brace, there would be no means to enable the trunk to de-rotate and achieve some rotational correction from the brace.

Can Cobb angle curves in the mid-30s progress after skeletal maturity is achieved?

Ms. Janssen: The progression of curves over 30° Cobb can and do occur and this information is well documented.

The most probable cause of curve progression after a person is skeletally mature is that they are used to being in the position of the scoliosis; therefore, that is where the body stays most of the time. The body is fixed in the uneven position from the scoliosis. If they don't have a strategy as to how to move themselves out of the curve in three dimensions, then they stay there. The tight tissues stay tight and those that have lengthened out to accommodate the curvature remain lengthened.

The mechanical forces, originating from the uneven load on the trunk from the curve, interacting with gravity and movements of daily life, slowly push the person more into the curve. This can happen slowly a little each day, week, or year, causing the spine to slowly collapse into the curve. This is more likely to happen in curves that exceed a certain Cobb angle. It is the vicious cycle model proposed by Ian Stokes.[5]

The following information is from a Scoliosis Research Society meeting in 1982 and is also quoted in Weinstein's textbook, *The Pediatric Spine*. The salient point is that curves with Cobb angles of more than 30° at skeletal maturity have a greater chance of progressing up to .5° a year, and curves that are from 50° to 75° have a chance of progressing up to 1° a year. This is, of course, when a patient does not have any specific exercise training to stabilize the curves.

To support this information further, Dr. Stu Weinstein outlines four growth factors and two curve factors that have big impact on predicting curve progression.

Growth Factors:

1. The younger the patient is at age of diagnosis.

2. Greater risk of progression before the onset of menarche in females.

3. The lower the Risser grade at curve detection, the greater the risk of progression.

4. Males are at 1/10 of the risk of progression than females, meaning curve progression is ten times more likely to occur in girls than boys.

Curve Factors:

1. Double curve patterns have greater tendency to progress than single.

2. The larger the magnitude of the curve at detection, the greater the risk of progression

Who is qualified to practice this specific type of treatment?
Ms. Janssen: We believe that a physical therapist certified in the Schroth Method is best qualified to practice the method. In addition, the prospective patient or a family member should ask the clinician when the physical therapist was certified, and how many scoliosis patients does this therapist treat annually. It is always best to seek a clinician who actively practices the method. Scoliosis Rehab Inc. with its certified instructors for the Barcelona Scoliosis Physiotherapy School trains and certifies physical therapists, under the direction of school founder Dr. Manuel Rigo.

What is involved in becoming certified? How do you find out if there are any certified Schroth therapists in your area?
Ms. Janssen: The qualifications to practice this method are a basic certification course with an exam at the end. The course is two weeks long. It involves lecture and lab time spent practicing the method. This certification is good for three years, and at that time, additional training is required to maintain the certification.

The Barcelona Scoliosis Physiotherapy School maintains an international list of all professionals who have been trained through the school.

You can visit them at www.bspts.net. You can also visit our website, www.scoliosisrehab.com, for a list of all the PTs whom we have trained.

Does your clinic accept insurance?

Ms. Campo: Yes. We are in network for many insurance companies across the U.S., as we have treated patients from forty states, as well as a handful of international patients.

References:

[1] C. Fusco, MD, F. Zaina, MD, S. Atanasio, PT, M. Romano, PT, A. Negrini, PT, and S. Negrini, MD, "Physical exercises in the treatment of adolescent idiopathic scoliosis: An updated systematic review," *Physiotherapy Theory and Practice* 27, no.1 (2011): 80-114.

[2] H.R.Weiss, S. Negrini, M. Rigo, et al., "Indications for conservative management of scoliosis (guidelines)," *Scoliosis Journal* (2006), 1:5, doi:10.1186/1748-7161-1-5.

[3] Martha Hawes, "The use of exercises in the treatment of scoliosis: An evidence-based critical review of the literature," *Pediatric Rehabilitation* 6, no. 3-4 (2003): 171-182.

[4] S. Otman, N. Kose, Y. Yakut, "The efficacy of Schroth's three-dimensional exercise therapy in the treatment of adolescent idiopathic scoliosis in Turkey," *Saudi Med J* 26, no.9 (2005):1429-35.

[5] Ian AF Stokes, R. Geoffrey Burwell and Peter H. Dangerfield, "Biomechanical spinal growth modulation and progressive adolescent scoliosis – a test of the 'vicious cycle' pathogenetic hypothesis: Summary of an electronic focus group debate of the IBSE," *Scoliosis* (2006), 1:16, doi:10.1186/1748-7161-1-16.

PART VI

PSYCHOLOGICAL SUPPORT AND GUIDANCE

Robin Stoltz, Licensed Clinical Social Worker

Learning from Adversity: Twist of Fate

The parents of our generation tend to have a major flaw. We want to (*over*)protect our kids. We run interference to make sure they don't experience any pain. We want them to be as comfortable as possible.

What we don't seem to understand is, the very act of overprotecting ends up promoting the opposite. By not allowing them to experience problems, they cannot learn necessary skills to work through life challenges. We end up placing our children at a disadvantage in life, making them dependent upon us to solve their problems. We are inadvertently telling them, "You are not equipped to deal with this. We need to do it for you because you are not competent."

What we really need to do instead is to allow our children to encounter difficulties and come up with their own ways of coping. The only way children can do that is by experiencing both defeat and success. Our job as parents is to help our children learn to navigate through their adolescence and not play interference. Scoliosis does just that for us; it takes away our control.

The day your child walks into middle school wearing their new brace, you feel totally helpless. I worried that my daughter would be teased and her heart would be broken because she would see that kids can be mean. I worried she wouldn't know how to respond if someone said something that made her feel uncomfortable. I felt self-conscious for her. I wanted to tell her to be careful, that children can be cruel.

Resilience is a trait that all parents
need to teach their children,
but one which requires the parent
to allow the child to experience
the pain of disappointment.

Coping is taught, learned, and experienced. I like to say to my kids, "Stuff happens; now we have to figure out how to deal with it." After all, how can you learn to "bounce back" if you've never experienced a setback? In an ironic "twist of fate," scoliosis represents a means to learn such lessons that will serve our children through many life challenges.

Scoliosis is a disease that presents our children with opportunities for personal growth and the development of new coping skills. Most of all, it can be an experience where they might witness themselves overcoming challenges and become more capable and self-confident than they were before they began their journey with scoliosis, but only if you let them.

Communication 101

For parents of kids with scoliosis, figuring out when to be firm or lenient can be a challenge during adolescence. My husband, Mike, and I struggled mightily with when and how firmly to discipline. Sometimes it is difficult to remain consistent when teens become adept at finding our vulnerabilities and pushing those buttons, especially when one of the buttons is guilt.

We found ourselves questioning our own judgment: "Was I too hard on her? After all, maybe she's feeling bad today about herself because of the brace. Did someone say something to make her feel bad? But then again, she mouthed off to me. If I ignore this, it gives her the message that the behavior is acceptable. When should we give her leeway?"

We didn't think it would be a good message to be easier on our daughter for behaviors that were not acceptable, simply because she has scoliosis. We always had to ask ourselves what it was that we were disciplining—frustration with her body image or poor behavior. It was the unacceptable behavior that we had to discipline, while finding a way to tell her to talk through her feelings.

Getting a teenager to talk isn't always an easy task. Here are some hints:

- *Ask open-ended questions, where the response can't be given in one-word answers, such as, "yes," "no," or "good."*

- *Spend time together outside of the house (shopping, dining).*

- *Talk aloud about things that might interest teens.*

Because you, as an adult, are in control in your house (or so it seems), taking your teen off-grounds equalizes the playing field. Leah was more inclined to talk when we weren't at home. You'll be surprised by the new information you might learn about your teen's life and you may not even have to ask. Try not to take your child's frustrations personally, use humor, be creative in your approach, and think outside of the box.

If none of that works, there's always counseling. My husband and I are both psychotherapists. Leah has watched me treat adolescents since she was old enough to sneak into my office area to meet them. Yet when it was her turn to be a teen, speaking with me was out of the question. She told me, "I don't do feelings." Silly me! But when she got so angry one night that she slammed my bedroom door breaking the mirror, it was time for intervention beyond what we could provide. She was making it clear that she needed help and all we needed to do was listen.

Driving to counseling was where she inadvertently taught me about "neutral." In the neutral setting of the car, she talked about her day and shared other thoughts. If I wasn't too intrusive, she might even share more.

That being said, you need to know your own child and how much is too much. For instance, if your child is withdrawing from social contact and activities, or crying with any frequency, it's time to intervene.

Seeking Support

Our experience has been that once a child/teen is involved with a group of peers who understand what they are dealing with, any sense of despair they may experience from feeling different will diminish. Contact your nearest support group and help your child get involved. Curvy Girls are located internationally and are there to help support you through this journey. Online support is also provided through the Curvy Girls website: www.curvygirlsscoliosis.com.

If, however, you find that your child/teen needs more than peer support, do not be afraid to seek professional advice. Seeking help does not imply that you did something wrong or failed your child. Nor does it mean that something is wrong with your child. The purpose of seeking professional advice is to help guide you and your child through difficult challenges in life. Common themes that the experience of scoliosis may complicate are body image issues, learning problems, and family circumstances.

Choosing a Mental Health Professional

If your child needs to speak with a mental health professional and you live in the United States, you may first want to contact your health insurance provider for explanation of benefits and referrals in your area. They can provide you with a list of licensed behavioral health professionals who specialize in treating children/teens. Your pediatrician can also refer you to a licensed clinician in your area. You may also ask friends and family if there is someone they can recommend.

When seeking psychotherapy or mental health care, it is important that the professional you choose have the proper training and licensing. In the United States, the professions that are licensed to treat mental health conditions include clinical psychologists, clinical social workers, mental health counselors, and psychiatrists. It is possible that in your state or country there may be other licensing requirements and professions that are certified to practice behavioral health care. Check the requirements in your state or country.

EPILOGUE

EPILOGUE

Curvy Girls Today

They've endured the shame of feeling different and isolated among their peers. They wore their brace up to twenty-three hours a day while living with the constant fear of needing spinal fusion surgery. Their diagnosis of scoliosis might have felt as if it took something away from them, but in the end, it gave each one a special gift.

Leah's story speaks to her resilience. How does a kid make sense of doing all the "right" things, only to end up having to face their ultimate fear? What could have been a tale of victimization, depression, and a teen's sense that it was the end of her world, became a story of triumph… and, ultimately, a gift for others.

Today, Leah is studying International Business and Communications at American University in Washington, D.C. She is involved in two local area Curvy Girls groups, continues to help start support groups around the world, as well as maintain an international web-based presence for girls with scoliosis (www.curvygirlsscoliosis.com). Presently, there are thirty-seven Curvy Girls groups located throughout the United States, Canada, South America, Australia and Europe.

Esther's congenital conditions and previous experiences with surgery made her and her family's scoliosis journey one of re-traumatization. It was ironic that it was Esther who told her mother to, "Suck it up!" Just as she did with her family, Esther teaches us about courage. As the Hebrew meaning of her name "star" implies, her bright smile shines and projects hope at every meeting.

Esther continues as an active member of the Curvy Girls, supporting girls who need to be braced, as well as those preparing for surgery. After nine years of bracing, Esther is finally being weaned out of her brace. Once brace-free, Esther plans to celebrate her accomplishments and go on an over-due shopping spree. When Esther graduates high school, she plans to attend Nassau Community College and major in Early Childhood Education.

Danielle's embarrassment over her body and her brace forced her to wear baggy sweatshirts. Her mature perspective allowed her to extract from her scoliosis experience newfound beliefs that she can apply later in life. She took her shame over having scoliosis and turned it into pride over being different.

Today, Danielle studies Early Childhood Education with a concentration in Human Development at SUNY Geneseo. While at college, Danielle's love for dance led her to become a member of the Orchesis Dance Club where she enjoys participating in student-choreographed dances. She is excited to be studying abroad in Ireland next fall.

Liv is bravely continuing her own struggle with scoliosis. She is very articulate about her fragile self-image. As a teenager, she experiences a wide range of feelings, from the devastating fears about rejection to the joys of acceptance. She describes the disclosure of her scoliosis as accidental, but like so many girls, her secret wish is that other girls will know and accept her.

Today, Olivia attends high school and is finally out of her brace. Because her curves are unstable, spinal fusion surgery may still be in her future. She has committed to practicing the Schroth Method.

Alyssa's embarrassment over her scoliosis was eroding her self-esteem and reinforcing her shyness. She finds relief in what she resists the most, revealing her secret. Ultimately, she finds strength in her scoliosis and wants to help other girls cope. She learns that she is stronger than she believed.

Today, Alyssa is attending Boston University and majoring in Speech Pathology. Her love for ice-skating continues; she is part of Boston University's synchronized skating team where she skates competitively. Alyssa has committed herself to the Schroth Method in order to learn how to live a healthier life with curves.

Danielle G.'s mental toughness helps her to prepare for the worst. She is steadfast in her beliefs and focus. When she found out the worst wasn't so terrible, she threw herself into helping other girls. She is determined to be a good role model for those facing surgery. Danielle won an essay contest in school about her challenges with scoliosis. She uses the winnings to make surgery baskets that she takes to Curvy Girls in the hospital.

Today, Danielle continues as an active member of the Curvy Girls Support Group. Both Danielle and her mom have begun a beautiful tradition of providing a basket of essential items for the girls who await surgery. These baskets have become the signature gift from our hearts, representing the importance of having a scoli-family support team.

Deanna had been with the group for over two years wearing her brace faithfully. She was one of a few girls who never complained about having to wear her brace. Deanna and her friends even named her brace, Claire. She dealt with her feelings by talking to friends and keeping a journal, as she learned to accept Claire. With great joy we clapped for Deanna when she became "successfully" brace-free. After a rash of girls having surgery following faithful brace wear, Deanna was truly free … so we thought.

Deanna learned that she required surgery despite her valiant efforts at bracing. The group was devastated, to say nothing of how she and her family felt. She cried the day she found out, wrote in her journal, and talked with friends and family, and ultimately accepted the course her life had taken at sixteen. Today, Deanna is graduating high school and is looking forward to attending Long Island University/C.W. Post Campus as a Music Education major

Jenna's favorite quote from Emily Giffin, "Sometimes the absolute last thing you want is the one thing you need," speaks to her resourcefulness and ability to find opportunity when faced with adversity. Despite her profound sense of loss when diagnosed with scoliosis, complicated by loss of friends and a panic disorder, she learns to rely on herself. Jenna's creativity becomes enhanced by turmoil when she immerses herself into a new challenge, designing clothes.

Today Jenna is a fashion design major at the prestigious Parsons New School for Design and has been climbing the intern ladder at Milly, Machesa, and Nanette Lepore. She aspires to be a designer, and maybe even have her own line one day. The talented Ms. Stern's fashion illustrations for bracewear are featured in our book.

Rachel's experience has taught her the meaning of determination. She challenged herself to do whatever she could to exceed her perceived limitations in order to keep her scoliosis at bay. She too wore her brace faithfully for two and a half years, yet when she was finally brace-free, her curve continued to progress. Her commitment and success turned her fears into setting and achieving her goals, while allowing this strength of determination to fuel her. This trait will serve her throughout life. Along the way, her mother came to accept that she couldn't protect her daughter from experiencing disappointment, but she could support her and connect her to critical resources through this journey.

Today, Rachel practices her Schroth exercises five days a week and actively promotes the Schroth Method within the medical community. She continues to lead the Long Island Curvy Girls group while Leah is away at college. Like her mentor, Leah, Rachel strives to make a difference in the life of every young girl she meets. She takes girls shopping for brace-worthy clothing and holds at-home Schroth demonstrations for families and the health care community. When Rachel graduates high school she plans to attend college and major in Community and Nonprofit Leadership.

It is our hope that the strength and courage exhibited in each girl will be a source of inspiration for young readers and their families.

Curvy Girls are triumphant and you can be too!

Final Thoughts

People don't understand how cruel scoliosis can be during pre-adolescence and adolescence. To be honest, we don't think a lot of people even know what scoliosis is. We certainly didn't. Too often, we've heard the remark, "It's not like you can die from it." While this is a good perspective for our families to maintain, what about the part of scoliosis that no one sees—the emotional impact on how our children view their bodies and feel about themselves. Because scoliosis happens most frequently during the years when fitting in is at the forefront of concern, scoliosis can quietly erode self-esteem and at times have devastating effects on our children's mental health.

Struggling alone with scoliosis changed with the advent of Curvy Girls peer-led support groups. It took one person to make the change. Just one. It's been nearly six years since Leah started Curvy Girls, and the ripple effect of this one act of kindness is still being felt. What evolved has inspired a growing mission and movement that the writers and their daughters have come to share.

Being a Curvy Girl has empowered our girls to deal with the challenges of scoliosis, as well as teaching them the power of giving back to their community. Standing as examples, they help each other while healing themselves. They learn to support each other through difficult times, as well as applaud accomplishments. As parents, we are proud as we watch our daughters grow into advocates for change.

As new Curvy Girls chapters start around the world, it's as if Leah is passing down her HALO award to each new girl, so that they can each pay forward the Curvy Girls mission of helping and leading others. You no longer have to be alone in this journey.

The members of our support groups have inspired us and have fueled our vision for change. Sociologist Margaret Read once wrote, "Never doubt that a small group of thoughtful, committed individuals can change the world; indeed, it's the only thing that ever has."

This is the message we live by, and it motivates us every day to provide a supportive forum for more girls and families, while we work towards implementing a permanent change in the standard of care for scoliosis.

Glossary
Words Every Parent Needs to Know

Apex measures the maximum point of the curve.

Asymmetry unevenness between parts of the body.

Bone Age determined with an x-ray of the left wrist and compared to chronological age.

Boston Brace the most commonly used TLSO brace; low profile made of lightweight plastic and padding usually worn between sixteen- to twenty-three-hours a day. Strategically placed pads apply pressure on the curve, and spaces are located opposite the areas of pressure.

Cervical Spine vertebrae C1-C7, located in the neck.

Charleston Bending Brace® a nighttime "bending brace" made of molded plastic and padding, worn only while sleeping; overcorrects by bending curve in opposite direction.

Cobalt Chrome Rod a type of metal that is used during spinal fusion surgery on bigger, stiffer curves.

Cobb Angle standard measurement of the spinal curve in scoliosis.

Compensatory Curve a curve that develops in response to the imbalance produced by the primary curve.

Formetric Scan a non-radiographic assessment of spinal deformity that uses surface topography to evaluate trunk shape.

Fusion when two bones become permanently joined.

Grafts shavings of bone or bone substitutes placed along vertebrae to aid in the spinal fusion process.

Growth Plate the area near the ends of all long bones in children and adolescents where cartilage slowly changes into bone. The growth plate is considered closed or ossified when there is no more cartilage remaining.

Idiopathic Scoliosis a spine curvature with no known cause.

Kyphosis excessive outward curvature in the upper thoracic spine causing a hunching.

Lordosis an inward curvature of the spine causing sway back.

Lumbar Spine vertebrae L1 to L5, located in the lower spine.

Milwaukee Brace a full-torso brace that extends to the base of the skull.

Molded Brace a brace made from plaster that is conformed to the person's body.

Orthotist with regard to scoliosis, an orthotist is a professional technician who custom makes back braces.

Ossify to harden, turn to bone.

Osteno Ostoma tumors that are an underlying condition that brings on scoliosis.

PCA Pump a device that lets the patient control the amount of intravenous pain medication received.

Providence Brace a low-profile plastic molded brace only worn while sleeping, provides similar correction to daytime braces for mild to moderate curvature

Rigo System Cheneau Brace (RSC)® a three-dimensional brace. Unlike most TLSOs, the RSC® brace is not full-contact; it does not touch the body everywhere. It reinforces the correction that people learn while doing Schroth exercises.

Risser Sign a grading system for ossification (hardening) of the cartilage of the iliac crest apophysis (growth plate located in the outer edge of the pelvis) which can be helpful in the prediction of scoliosis curve progression; Risser 4: complete ossification without fusion; Risser 5: fusion of the ossified apophysis to the ilium, representing growth is complete.

Scoliometer a screening device used to measure distortions of the torso.

Scoliosis a musculoskeletal disease that causes lateral curvature of the spine of 10° or more, resulting in a spine that appears S- or C-shaped rather than straight.

ScoliScore® prognostic genetic test which analyzes the DNA from a saliva swab of patients diagnosed with adolescent idiopathic scoliosis. The results of the test range from 1-200, indicating potential for progression by low, medium, or high.

Section 504 School systems abide by this section of the Federal Rehabilitation Act of 1973 that guarantees certain rights to persons with disabilities.

Skeletal Maturity when bones and spine are finished growing

SpineCor® System soft TLSO made from cloth and elastic corrective straps used in low to moderate immature curves. Assists in retraining body posture for self-correction of the scoliosis curves. This brace must be worn for twenty hours a day.

Spondylolisthesis the forward slip out of position of one vertebra on another that can cause pain. Once diagnosed certain activities and sports should be modified or stopped in order to prevent further movement. Gymnastics, weight training, and football are several activities that put a greater amount of stress on the lower vertebrae in the spine.

Spondylolysis the actual defect or fracture in the posterior part of the vertebrae that allows a spondylolisthesis to occur.

Stainless Steel Rod alternative to the cobalt chrome rod, used in spinal fusion surgery with larger more aggressive curves.

Syrinx a collection of cerebral spinal fluid within the spinal cord, often resulting in scoliosis.

Tanner Stages the measurement of secondary sex characteristics (e.g., breast bud, genitals, pubic hair, facial hair).

Thoracic Spine vertebrae T1 to T12 located in the mid- to upper-spine.

Titanium Rod a metal device used to correct the curvature of scoliosis in spinal fusion surgery; works well on small, less rigid curves.

TLSO Brace lightweight plastic spinal brace that provides key pad placement, putting three-point pressure on the curve to support the thoracic, lumbar, and sacral regions of the spine.

Triradiated Cartilage hip growth plate. An open cartilage indicates growth is not over; a closed cartilage is an indication that growth is complete.

Vertebrae bones that make up the spinal column.

Vertebral Body Stapling A surgical procedure where staples are inserted on the convex (outer) side of the curve with the intent of preventing the opposite side from progressing. The criteria for this procedure include spine flexibility, curves less than 40° and years of growth remaining.

Acknowledgments

We have a saying in Curvy Girls, "If you've made a difference in one person's life, you've done a great thing." Our journey to helping girls and families like us who are profoundly affected by scoliosis was enriched by people similarly driven to go the "extra mile" to help others. We extend our gratitude to our contributors and advisors who are committed to making a difference:

- Alyssa and Jeanne, Esther and Sheryl, Danielle and Susan, Danielle and Debbie, Olivia and Judith, Deanna and Marianne, Jenna and Patrice, and our daughters Leah and Rachel—a heartfelt thank you for allowing us to share your stories to help other girls and families to never feel alone.
- Our own Curvy Girl, Ms. Jenna Stern, for all the hours spent sketching our fashion illustrations. Your talent is a true gift to this project.
- Curvy Girl Dana Fauth for her insightful photograph portraying the essence of the Curvy Girl experience.
- Curvy Mom Patrice Stern for her commitment, time and talents.
- Our Long Island Curvy Girls' families who taught us the true value of support. You were our inspiration for writing this book.
- Dr. John Labiak, Dr. Laurence Mermelstein, and Dr. Stefano Negrini for generously offering their time and medical expertise to educate our readers on the U.S. and European approaches to the treatment of scoliosis.
- Orthotists Mike Mangino and Steve Mullins for the patience and empathy they provide all our Curvy Girls when putting put on that first brace.
- Orthotist Grant Wood for his dedication to the field of conservative treatment and contribution to three-dimensional bracing.
- Raul Fuentes for sharing his radiological expertise and the care he takes with each child.

- Robyn Rexford, the reason Curvy meetings are soda- and sugar-free, for sharing her common sense approach to nutrition ensuring healthier bodies for our children as they grow.
- Dr. Michael Vitale for his ongoing support of all our Curvy endeavors.
- Patrick Knott is deeply appreciated for sharing his expertise and guidance whenever needed.
- Curvy Mom Patty Borzner for sharing her own lessons learned.
- Beth Roach for her recovery tips and friendship when arranging to be Leah's PICU nurse. It meant the world to both of us.
- Tara Mulvaney, Glenn Campbell, and Seth Schwartz who took the time to find the answers and help us with legal matters.
- Tom Emmerson from Alternative Graphic Solutions for his talents and commitment. In this world there are no accidents. When Tom contacted Curvy Girls for his daughter Rachel, we had no idea the impact we would have on each other. Your support and talents have been invaluable in helping us pass along the message.
- Editor Doug Love for treading gently but skillfully.
- Grammatical gratitude goes to David Schwartz, Diane Schwartz, and Michael Stoltz.
- Paige McCoy for her talent in photo-journaling Smithtown High School HALO surprise.
- To the staff at Scoliosis Rehab for always greeting our families with warm hugs as if they were long lost family members.

The African proverb, "It takes a whole village to raise a child," rings true when we think about our village of supporters who encouraged Leah's idea and helped her to believe in herself.

- Sharon Vigliarolo, Lori Gerrard, and Mae Caime for making sure Curvy Girls happened.
- Karen Correia, PT, for introducing Leah to Rachel, her very first Curvy Girl.

- Caring Long Island Spine Specialists' staff up front and behind the scenes who continue to support Curvy Girls.
- Leah's surgeon, Dr. Mermelstein, who led us gracefully and confidently through this journey.

There are people in this world who use their skills and talents for the betterment of others. Serving as role models for our girls, they set a standard for future generations to make a difference in this world:

- We admire Dr. Oheneba Boachie-Adjei for his living philosophy that "medicine is a privilege and not a right." Your selfless service to those in need serves as an inspiration to Curvy Girls around the world. Join Dr. Boachie and his FOCOS team and make a difference (www.orthofocos.org).
- Always at the forefront of change, a special acknowledgment to Joe O'Brien, President, CEO and Patient, National Scoliosis Foundation (www.scoliosis.org) for being a catalyst in the growth of Curvy Girls beyond Long Island. When Nickelodeon was looking for a HALO recipient, Joe connected them with Leah. NSF has been advocating for early detection and treatment for over thirty years while educating, encouraging and empowering patients.
- For their vision in bringing the Schroth Method to the United States and their expertise shared in our book, we are grateful to Beth Janssen and Rhonda Campo. Their dedication and passion to help ALL generations affected with scoliosis is a true testament to who they are. Beth, you put the light back in our children's eyes and provide them with tools to help them live a pain free life with scoliosis. On behalf of all the Curvy Girls and their families, thank you both for continuing to help bring forth a change in the care of this disease.
- To our honorary Curvy Girl, JoEllen Hegmann, whose dedication to raising awareness and hard work with the Scoliosis Association of Long Island has improved the quality of life for people living with scoliosis. We admire and respect all that you have done. Thank you for always looking out for our Girls.

- Justin Timberlake has used his talents to make a difference in children's lives. When you chose Leah as your HALO recipient, curvy girls all over the country watched and no longer felt alone.
- Nick Cannon's vision of having a celebrity select and award teens for "helping and leading others" continues to inspire kids all over the country.
- Josh Wright, Pete Wilkinson, Maggie Wang, Lauren Lazin, Bronwen O'Keefe and the TeenNick staff whose talents enabled hundreds of girls to take action in their community culminating in the first Curvy Girls International Convention.

And then there are those that stand by quietly supporting us, allowing us to dare greatly to achieve our dreams:

Our children, Paul and Leah Stoltz, and Tara, Joseph, Brittney, and Rachel Mulvaney for putting up with our all-consuming days and nights of living on the computer.

To my own mom, Zelda, who showed me the path of resilience and told me I could accomplish whatever I wanted no matter my challenge.

We hit the lottery with husbands, Bobby Mulvaney and Michael Stoltz, whose love and encouragement over these past few years is what helped us through those twelve-hour days of writing and editing. It was your undying support that allowed us to remain focused and ultimately achieve our goal. Always and Forever.

And finally, to all those impacted with scoliosis we hope that by sharing our personal stories we have helped you feel less alone. Together, let us continue to make a difference.

About the Authors

Theresa E. Mulvaney

The mother of four children ages seventeen to twenty-seven. Theresa has been a parent advocate for children with learning disabilities and their families, as well as her current work for those affected by scoliosis. Her advocacy to protect the rights of special education children resulted in a favorable decision from the Commission of Education preventing the local school district from unilaterally removing an entire group of special education students from their home school without their parents' consent.

More recently, her daughter's experience with scoliosis and their leadership roles with Curvy Girls have prompted Theresa to advocate for modifying the U.S. standard of care for scoliosis to emphasize more conservative approaches.

Theresa and her husband, Bobby, an electronics engineering IT professional, reside in Mount Sinai, N.Y.

Robin Machson Stoltz, LCSW, BCD, CASAC

An educator and clinical social worker for over 30 years, Robin is also the mother of two young adult children. Her younger child Leah's experience with scoliosis, which inspired her to start Curvy Girls, also led Robin to meet with Girls' parents to lend comfort and guidance to their plight. After many years as Deputy Executive Director of a behavioral health center, Robin now has a private practice specializing in adolescents and adults. She holds credentials in addiction disorders and has recently completed advanced training in EMDR, an evidence-based approach to helping people overcome trauma-involved experiences. Robin is currently completing her second book addressing the experience of paternal abandonment.

Robin and her husband, Michael, also a social worker, reside in Smithtown, N.Y.

STRAIGHT TALK
WITH THE
CURVY GIRLS

To order additional copies of this book
and make arrangements for
Authors and Curvy Girls speaking engagements:
www.straighttalkscoliosis.com

www.curvygirlsscoliosis.com